In Dire Straits

Keeping Spirit Alive When the Wheels Come Off

Jim Currie

Savant Books and Publications
Honolulu, HI, USA
2011

Published in the USA by Savant Books and Publications
2630 Kapiolani Blvd #1601
Honolulu, HI 96826
http://www.savantbooksandpublications.com

Printed in the USA

Edited by Alice Sullivan
Cover and Interior Illustrations by Jim Currie
Cover Photo courtesy of J. Eric Smith
Cover Design by Daniel S. Janik

13-digit ISBN:978-0-9845552-9-1
10-digit ISBN:0-9845552-9-3

This work is a topical memoir. The author has tried to make the
information in this book as accurate as possible; however, some
names have been changed to protect the identity of specific
individuals and institutions. Furthermore, the information conveyed
was current only up to the date that the manuscript went into
production and is presented strictly from the author's point of view.
Therefore, this work should be used only as a general inspirational
guide not as an authoritative or reliable source of medical or
historical information.

Dedication

To Myra, with the greatest appreciation for your support in my darkest hours, and whose creative insights on healing, personal and planetary, always spurred a deeper level of exploration.

Acknowledgment

So many people played an important role in the creation of this book. I wouldn't have had the strength to write it without the help of my good friend Myra, Ralph Golan, M.D, David Bove, N.D., Thomas Brown, M.D., Trevor Marshall Ph.D., Carol Nicholson, and other healers, including a good number of honeybees and a brown lab named Bella.

Satish Kumar and Larry Dossey were quick to add a helping hand in reviewing chapters, and both provided a standard for the kind of thoughtful, idea-rich writing that I aspired to in creating the book. They along with Howard Zinn also fortified the premise that personal and planetary healing share similarities, and can provide insights to one another in finding a healing path.

Much thanks to Dan Janik and Alice Sullivan at Savant for close attention to details and shepherding the book through the editing and publication process. You saw mistakes and omissions that I missed and supported the idea that art was as important to this book as words.

Others who added a dose of spirit, laughter, or strategically-positioned shot of bee venom included Darrell Duffey, Mel Walters, Chris Merritt, Ph.D., Charlyn Golan, Barbara Deal, and the many Friends of Sydney's Thumb.

I'm particularly indebted to Sky Carpenter, Henry Miller, Myra, and Gigi for imparting the imperative to paint and create as long as there is breath, a glint of light, and energy to lift a pen or paintbrush. From all of you I learned the secrets of turning inflammation into curiosity, determination, discovery, and occasionally something wonderful.

Contents

In Dire Straits

"To be hopeful in bad times is not just foolishly
romantic. It is based on a fact that human history is a
history not only of cruelty but also of compassion,
sacrifice, courage, kindness. And if we do act in
however small a way, we don't have to wait for some
grand utopian future. The future is an infinite
succession of presents, and to live now as we think
human beings should live in defiance of all that is bad
around us is itself a marvelous victory."

—Howard Zinn

Introduction

In February 1998, I lost my mom to non-Hodgkin's lymphoma in a wrenching ordeal at Cheswicke Hopital. The two of us had always been close and her death opened up a great whirlpool in my path that swallowed me whole. I found myself retreating from family and friends and avoiding commitments of any sort. I was dazed and exhausted. I'm sure that if a dive team had been able to find me and monitor my vital signs, they would have been hard pressed to detect pulse, reflexes, and signs of consciousness. I guess I didn't realize how much I would miss her and how hard it would be to recover.

As a person long interested in integral psychology and Eastern spirituality, I knew there was no mystery about what I was going through. My grief reflected more than the loss of someone dear, but a deeper despair and attachment that needed attention. For several months, I worked on this with an awareness that this kind of healing was something you didn't rush. I needed time to forget and dull some of the most acute pain, time to cry the tears of frustration over what had happened, time to my divert attention and energy toward work or whatever it was that I was faking on my weekday hours, time to accept the reality that my phone calls home would no longer be answered, and time to spout my still eruptive anger over the backward medical system I felt was responsible for so many mindless mistakes in my mom's last two weeks. Then maybe after all this emotion had worked its way through my over-wrought mind and body, just maybe I would pop to the surface like a cork released from a sunken ship.

I didn't exactly pop to the surface, but in summer of 1998, I was at least becoming more functional at work and more sociable around friends. On at least a few occasions, I laughed and told a bad joke or two. I even spent some time with a comedian and impressionist friend named Duffey who was hoping to land an engagement in Vegas. For some reason he figured that I was just the one to help him create a bomb-proof routine for an upcoming audition. His misplaced confidence in me had only slightly eroded when I offered up a candid confession: "Duff, I would really like to help you with your material, but you need to understand one thing: I'm not really a funny guy."

"Yes!" he declared emphatically. This was the gold-plated theme he was looking for—a shaky comedian whose material was being composed by a humorless and morose mortician. He was sure it would turn him into a headliner on the Strip.

In the fall he headed off to Vegas without his personal mortician and I took an extended leave from work to travel through Europe. After a few rough spots, my spirit enlivened and so, too, my *joie de vivre*.

Six months after I returned to Seattle, my health took a strange turn. The fatigue I had been struggling with for over a year suddenly intensified, and then, out of the blue, my fingers and toes swelled up, making walking and any kind of athletic activity near-impossible. Although I didn't know it at the time, I was in the early throes of an aggressive immune system rebellion in which my own joints and connective tissue were being targeted by T-cells and inflammatory cytokines. I seemed caught up in various scenes from *The Fantastic Voyage*, except there was no Raquel Welch in her prime to rescue me.

Oliver Sacks, the renowned medical doctor and author of *Awakenings*, once noted that nothing illuminates the human condition like disease. My own ordeal from 1998 onward sensitized me to my own vulnerability and prompted deeper reflection. Suddenly freedom and mobility were at stake, and increasingly, my personal identity because sports, physical activity, and footloose backpacking were so important to me. Coming to grips with this changed my perspective on what I valued, what I believed in, who was most important in my life, and what I really needed to devote my energies to. This disease would also simultaneously tax all my rational problem-solving abilities, sense of humor, and spiritual balance.

Soon after September 11, 2001, it dawned on me that the stress and dis-ease that I had been experiencing were now being felt by the country as a whole. In both cases, the stealthy attacker had delivered a telling blow and receded into the darkness, leaving a wake of turmoil and uncertainty. The challenge was to find a measured and mindful response rather than lash out reflexively at some vague evil.

While the country was muddling through its identification of friend and foe, searching for credible voices of authority, and mobilizing for retaliation, I was negotiating the labyrinth of a disordered and fragmented medical system that couldn't have been designed any worse to handle a disease like my own. It was clear that I needed to adopt an alternative approach, maybe even a guerrilla mentality, or I was going to be a casualty of neglect like so many other people with severe chronic diseases that cross into several medical disciplines. I was equally determined to avoid off-the-shelf cures that only promised complications more dire than the disease itself.

As it turned out, many of the curiosities awakened by a liberal education suddenly became relevant to my difficulties. These included studies in modern art, the great ideas in Western civilization, Eastern philosophy, cognitive and integral psychology, and the great breakthroughs in science and technology. Each offered important instruction in creative problem solving. They also fortified me with conviction that I was capable of being my own healer, or at least co-healer, and needn't be simply powerless, accepting pills, IVs and injections that I had little confidence in.

Early on, I arrived at an intriguing proposition: the possibility that I might benefit from the open and exploratory mindset I practiced in my many backpacking trips through Europe. I had always tried to remain mindful and present in the moment. I expected complication, and when I encountered it I tried to treat it with the light-heartedness that the French writer, Rabelais, suggested when he declared, "For all your ills, I give you laughter."

In each of my trips I encountered bumps in the road and impediments, but these always seemed to elicit resourcefulness and creativity. As a result, I almost always felt stronger and better able to deal with future difficulties. Perhaps it was possible to bring that same attitude to my current traumas, though a considerable percentage of my waking hours was spent soaking in a bathtub or retreating to bed from complete exhaustion.

Testing this idea led me down many new and strange alleyways. In short order, I was working my way through an inner Marais and arriving at an interior opera, rich with drama and enchantment. In many ways the people, creatures, and discoveries would rival my best finds in travel to Venice, Paris, Western Ireland, and Upper Bavaria. These included the following Quixotic foibles, edifying dramas, and synchronicities: the bridge with no visible means of support; an intuitive brown lab with a nose for miraculous cures; a wild man floating down the Rhine on a hospital gurney; Jack Nicholson and Faye Dunaway making a return to Chinatown; stings of awareness from a horde of bees; and a bear that can materialize a soluble fish.

In each case, the discoveries either answered an important health or spiritual question or pointed me down an illuminating path. No Eurail Pass was required, no airline ticket to London, no loge tickets to the Paris Opera. It was not even necessary to have a sturdy set of legs, an agile set of hands, or a completely defogged brain. The only real necessity was a commitment to playfulness and imagination and a refusal to be contracted and plundered by pain and fear.

Buddhists have long expressed the view that life difficulty, friction, and chaos represent an opportunity for spiritual growth. Buddhist masters are even noted for congratulating their students in the midst of their grief and suffering because they now have the chance to sweep away the heavy dust of old karma. In the same tradition, I compassionately congratulate you for landing at the doorstep of whatever life difficulty you have been presented with. Open the grand door before you with broom in hand, offer up a good laugh at the surprise, absurdity, or tragic irony, then enter into the mansion with a furious brushstroke and a lighthearted imagination. In the process you may discover that the feathery spirit can rise above the anxieties, pain, and suffering of the world.

Chapter 1

I'll Leave You Alone to Digest the News

"A bump in the road, a minor setback," I murmured to myself as I waited in Seattle's Minor Medical Clinic to see a rheumatologist about my swollen foot and right ring finger. The room was packed like an Italian train station and none of the trains seemed to be running. Finally, a name was called and a crippled lady was escorted into one of the waiting rooms. All around me people breathed sighs of relief. I ran a quick inspection—most of these people were elderly and in pretty bad shape, wearing braces, bandages, or relegated to wheel chairs. I turned toward my invisible friend and long-time travel companion from Bodh Gaya, India, and was chagrined to see that he had wandered off.

"Figures," I murmured. Left me in the lurch again—just like that night in Interlaken when I was locked out of the youth hostel and nearly froze to death. Luckily, my wits were about me and I discovered that I could prevent hypothermia by taking refuge in a lavatory and wrapping myself in five rolls of toilet paper—nature's finest insulator. Now there was mindfulness in practice, mindfulness under duress that would

7

have impressed the Dalai Lama and maybe even Buddha himself.

I decided to fall into emptiness meditation—a perfect practice for dealing with all manner of human bottleneck: train station snafus, waiting room back-ups, and airliners stuck in holding patterns. Closing my eyes, I took several deep breaths, but rather than floating in a warm ocean, I found myself on a bullet train streaking for Paris. Now this was a fantasy I could get into. Paris is exactly where I wanted to be.

When I broke out of the reverie, I noticed an octogenarian in a wheel chair at the far end of the room. She was chirping about her beloved husband now dead and buried. She appeared to be alone, but I knew that wasn't so. My food-challenged, Indian friend was there with her, hearing her out, intoning assurance and offering comfort. It was just like him to find someone like her struggling with fear, constantly turning pain into suffering, and to try to help them allay the worry.

I guess I didn't rate. No major suffering here, no dark night of the soul. Just a damn painful foot and a ballooning digit. Maybe after my appointment I would exaggerate my condition to curry his sympathy. I would take it to the hilt—tell him that Doc Reece said amputation might be necessary and that this might affect walking and backpacking.

Yes, that was the perfect angle of attack—no more backpacking and hiking. It meant as much to my friend as it did to me—an attachment he couldn't deny. We had been traveling together for six years now. In Europe we trekked through the high Alps, negotiated the perils of romance with a wild German rose in Berchtesgaden, and even collaborated on a book about travel and Eastern philosophy, entitled, *The Mindful Traveler: A Guide to Journaling and Transformative Travel*. If this Buddha suffered any attachment, it was certainly footloose travel.

The nurse called my name and a mere hour later, Dr. Reece was examining me closely. He didn't seem to be having a good day—no cheer whatsoever. He asked a few perfunctory questions about first symptoms and I blathered on about a pneumonia incident in Denmark and extreme fatigue that set in after my mom's death a year-and-a-half earlier. He mostly seemed to be focused on my nails, staring at them like a coroner inspecting a fresh corpse showing a most interesting pathology.

"And these? Always had problems with this kind of discoloration?"

"Yes, but aside from being an eyesore, they never caused any problems. I figured I might have some kind of allergy or yeast problem."

"Any psoriasis?"

"Nope."

He paused thoughtfully, a zippered look fixed on his face. "I'm sorry my friend, but you have psoriatic arthritis." The sentence ended with the finality of an obituary.

I shrugged dismissively and he replied, "I'll leave you alone to absorb the news." He handed me a thick medical book on rheumatological disorders and retired.

I turned to the marked pages and was shocked by a series of gruesome hands and fingers, then paged to a section on feet more birdlike than human—gnarled and mutilated that could have belonged to the gargoyles of Notre Dame or Lourdes. That wasn't the end of it. Another section was devoted to deformed knees, twisted backs, and displaced shoulder joints. Quasimodo, the Hunchback of Notre Dame. Was it possible that this was my future as well? I couldn't bear to look and paged quickly to the treatment section.

It wasn't very hopeful. Prednisone was used selectively to control swelling, but because it was a corticosteroid, was not recommended for long-term use. The focus of treatment was modulating the immune system, lessening the T-cell assault on connective tissue. Nothing had proved very effective. In past years, gold salts were used extensively, but in recent decades, the drug of choice was methotrexate.

"Methotrexate?" I blurted out. That was one of the main drugs used to treat my mom's lymphoma. Along with prednisone and Vincristine it had quickly destroyed her immune system. Six weeks of methotrexate had landed her in critical care where she died of Hospital Pneumonia, that antibiotic-resistant disease that hospitals don't really want to talk about. I was suddenly awash in memories of her last days in which I had become her twenty-four-hour helper. It was a futile and exasperating effort, compounded by one mistake after another by the staff at Cheswicke Hospital.

"No way," I murmured.

The doctor returned and began talking in formal jargon but my attention was fleeting. I guess I was having a little trouble absorbing the news. I focused long enough to hear him say something to the effect that methotrexate was the best bet for keeping the disease in check and allowing me to live a near-normal life.

"I don't think we'll be buying into that program," I answered.

"Some other drugs will soon be coming out, but right now this is the best option." He reached for a pen, scribbled out the prescription, and left me alone.

I gathered my possessions, left the prescription behind, and limped down the hall toward the exit. A few minutes later, I passed into a rain-driven street and stared up the hill at the main tower of Cheswicke Hospital, veiled in low-lying fog. My heartbeat quickened and I became flushed with the residue of unwanted memories, a feeling of futile desperation in trying to save my mom's life two years earlier. I breathed a heavy sigh and the hospital seemed to recede in the mist, reminding me of a dreamy Monte Cassino or the cloaked monasteries of Mycenae. A distant traveler might even imagine it secreted some higher knowledge, perhaps the arcane practice of hermetic cognoscenti. And yet it was closer to the opposite—a citadel of positivism.

Whatever prejudices I might have about it, I had to admit that it was still about the best hospital in the city, and maybe the Pacific Northwest. And yet I somehow knew that at this very moment any number of major breakdowns were brewing—overburdened doctors and nurses working off different protocols, staff that didn't speak English as a first language, and perhaps an outbreak of killing pneumonia linked to uncontrolled staph bacteria. I wouldn't be at all surprised to learn that three patients were unaccounted for, the west wing was being quarantined, and a ragged-looking phlebotomist was out on the roof trying to talk down a disconsolate psychiatrist. The systems had simply run amok.

Ironically, here I was, two years later at an associated clinic, being advised to take methotrexate and prednisone and trust in the system. Was this mere coincidence or was I being manipulated by some disembodied force with a very bad sense of humor? I reached my car and Buddha was already inside, apparently apprised of the news. "I guess I knew it could be something serious."

He didn't answer, but I could sense his sympathy and concern.

"There's got to be a way to solve this. After all, we've been in some pretty tight situations before. In our trips there was always a way out of every debacle." He seemed to be giving me his full attention.

"Remember when we got pneumonia outside of Aarhus? I thought we were cooked—*finis*, candidates for an apple in the mouth—but we survived. Relied on rest, prana breathing, and mega-doses of bee pollen."

I closed my eyes and took a deep breath. For a few seconds I felt only emptiness, and then it occurred that all this was only an illusion, arising out of unfounded anxiety. None of it was substantial. I simply needed to step out of the dense field of self-created nightmare. Unfortunately, my throbbing right foot jolted me back. All I could think about was dropping into a soothing tub and cranking the Jacuzzi to full.

Kung Fu was the first major TV series to introduce Eastern philosophy to a western audience. The main character was Kwai Chang Caine, a fugitive Shaolin monk wandering barefoot through the Wild, Wild West.

Caine's introduction to the locals was minimally humble: "My name is Caine. I have come to help." Trouble was, except for the downtrodden and suffering, most of the locals viewed him as a trespasser and trouble-maker. Every time he would come to the aid of a Chinese railroad coolie, scarlet-lettered whore, or refugee, he would antagonize the biggest ranchers, craven mine owners and railroad bosses, or the corrupt sheriff who did their bidding.

A man of peace, Caine would always try to avoid violence but his prospects were no more promising than Arjuna in the *Bhagavad Gita*. Forced into a corner, he would turn into a whirling dervish, smiting his attackers with a blizzard of thrusts, chops, and acrobatic kicks.

What I enjoyed most, however, was Caine's economy of action, always grounded in Eastern philosophy. He relied heavily on metaphors of tigers and dragons, monkeys and crafty birds, and always found a way to use the energies of an evil adversary against him—the high art of *wu-wei* (loosely translated as letting go and non-striving). Caine was the master of energy transformation and spiritual balance.

I wondered if *wu-wei* held the key to my own healing. No doubt, my own *chi* had been at an all-time low since my trauma at Cheswicke Hospital. I had suffered extreme fatigue from the ordeal that included many nights without sleep both before and after my mom's death. An acupuncturist had even told me that my several pulses were "extremely stringy," whatever that meant.

Kwai Chang Caine was as much a healer as a martial

13

artist. His only possession was a small brown pouch that contained his talisman and an assortment of Chinese herbs that could salve wounds, tonify organs, and fortify his own chi. On more than a few occasions he used them to perform a miracle cure.

I didn't have a little brown bag full of roots and rhizomes but I did have a helper of my own. My best friend Madeleine, an inveterate reader, had made a lifelong avocational study of alternative medicine. She had been by my side during the ordeal at Cheswicke, helping me to avert most of the mistakes of the inattentive staff. In the year that followed, she helped me with my eruptive anxieties and occasional panic. She would have accompanied me to the clinic except that I told her I could manage on my own—no sense in having her miss work for someone else's doctor appointment. Besides, I knew that the serene spiritual one would be with me, unless he got distracted by someone who was really suffering.

Madeleine had long believed in the idea that healing was an inside job and that anyone with a reasonably analytical mind could become an able self-healer. Over the years from our many conversations about healing, I had decided that this was an important aspect of higher self or Buddha nature. In my travel book, published in 2000, it was Madeleine I was really thinking of when I suggested the *Credo and Curiosities of Buddha as Healer*.

The credo related to helping others as well as self. It recognized the many interactions between mind, body, and spirit. These included the positive influence of joy, love, and purpose on physiology, as well as the corresponding negative effects of gloom, fear, and lack of meaning. The influence worked in other ways as well, for example, physical well-being on mind and spirit.

Credo and Curiosities of Buddha as Healer

Credo and Mindset
1. I can monitor my own health and find ways to optimize wellness.
2. I can make changes necessary to correct imbalances and to heal myself.
3. In order to heal others I may have to heal myself.
4. Caring, love, and compassion promote wellness and healing.

Questions and Curiosities
1. How is the mind/body system operating?
2. What are the pathways by which imbalances manifest as disease?
3. What are my personal weaknesses, vulnerabilities, and tendencies toward imbalance?
4. What signs and signals can I rely on to monitor my own health and wellness?
5. What capacities and functions are degraded by fatigue or stress?
6. How can I fortify myself to prevent illness?
7. What problems are beyond me and require the help of others?
8. How can I support and help others?

Source: *The Mindful Traveler* (Open Court, 2000)

I waited until evening to call Madeleine and fill her in on my appointment. She didn't know much about psoriatic arthritis, only related disorders such as rheumatoid arthritis, lupus, and fibromyalgia. When I described the pictures in the medical book, she answered that these might simply represent the extreme—"Medical texts are notorious for that."

Although concerned, she was upbeat and optimistic. "Now at least we have something to work with instead of just guessing. I'm sure there are non-toxic options to methotrexate."

Two hours later we were still on the phone, going through our combined libraries on healing and wellness, working back and forth between causes and effects and the limited information we had on remedies. The best idea we came up with was to put Ralph Golan on the case. He was a Seattle M.D. with a specialty in internal medicine whom both of us had visited for second opinions when a problem seemed beyond the expertise of our primary-care doctors. (He had opted out of the insured medical system and worked on his own.)

His healing philosophy was captured in an unusual book called *Optimal Wellness* that gave readers a fuller view of the physiological origins of disease and wellness. Unlike so many health books that were organized around diseases, their diagnosis and treatments, *Optimal Wellness* illuminated the pathways and the common denominators of illness, giving patients the tools to become their own healers or at least co-healers.

The book didn't specifically address psoriatic arthritis, but discussed immune-system stressors, their effects on different metabolic pathways, and how to reverse imbalances through herbs, diet, and life-style changes. My appointment was a few weeks later.

Ralph's office seemed to fit well with his reputation as an independent doctor drawing upon naturopathy, Eastern, and Western allopathic medicine. I was greeted at the door by a friendly brown lab named Bella who immediately urged me to help her destroy the latest edition of *Conde Nast*. She finished it off by twisting it against my resistance and I settled in a comfortable chair.

It was a pleasant, uncrowded environment, the kind of place you wouldn't mind visiting even if you weren't in the middle of a health crisis. The colors were warm and soothing and the walls tastefully adorned with interesting paintings of mountains and forests, each composition possessing a unique mood and spirit of place. This was such stark contrast to the moonbeam and angel art that so often covered the walls of energy healers and naturopaths.

Ralph greeted me wearing pressed canvas pants, an L.L. Bean chamois shirt, and a new pair of Ecco shoes. His voice was flat and monotone but his eyes were curious and alive.

He didn't seem to remember me from a previous appointment three years earlier. I filled him in quickly on my situation and immediately had the sense that we were operating at the same basic cadence—pianissimo.

He interrupted on two occasions to inspect my hands and feet but gave me a non-verbal clue to continue. I finished with my back history, then shifted to describe my appointment with Dr. Reece.

"Yes, I wouldn't dispute the diagnosis, but I'm sure there are some options here. I am no specialist. You need to understand that."

I nodded. "Yes, but you are a systems person. You make connections and that's the kind of thinking I can relate to."

He seemed flattered. He promptly jotted out a list of herbs that should reduce my inflammation—curcumin, boswellia, ginger, oregano, green tea, and willow. "Of course, these only deal with symptoms and it's important to treat the underlying imbalance. This is where there can be disagreement."

"What is causing the inflammation—a runaway immune system, or maybe something more fundamental?"

"Exactly. It's a matter of levels and point of origin. Why did the immune system suddenly go into overdrive and exactly what part?" He pedaled across his office to a stack of journal articles. "Read this paper and tell me what you think. I haven't really had the time to digest it, but it does suggest a radically different approach. It's about mycoplasma—a microbe that might start the process in motion. While you're looking into this, I'll do some background work. In a week or so we'll put our heads together again."

He shook my hand, then grasped my shoulder with genuine concern. He wanted me to know that he wasn't just sending me off to fend for myself, but that a partnership had been struck. This was just the kind of help I had been hoping for—an engaged doctor who valued my input and expected me to use my own mind and energy to help solve the problem at hand.

Chapter 2

Sleuthing

I guess I've always been drawn to radical ideas and unconventional voices. My personal library includes the novels of Henry Miller, Howard Zinn's *A People's History of the United States*, the most provocative novels of Gunter Grass, the mystical musings of Newton, the heretical reflections of Meister Eckhardt, the Gnostic Gospels, Stuart Wilde's writings on the wisdom of the Mongol warriors, the transcendental poetry of Blake, art of the great Luminists, and any number of political manifestos by Gore Vidal, Norman Mailer, Jean Breton, and Eugene Debs. Prime space is allocated to Golan's *Optimal Wellness*. If you give it close scrutiny, you realize that it fits the list. It is to medicine what the beliefs of the Albigensian heretics were to the Catholic Church, what the writings of de Sade and Rousseau were to the *Ancien Regime*, what the muckrakers were to meatpackers and nineteenth-century industrialists.

It is a subdued and subtle subterfuge camouflaged by a thicket of information about the workings of liver and pancreas, heart and kidneys, immune system and digestion, and the myriad connections between them. Golan gives you a full blow-up of the diagnostic box, and maybe in your inspection of it you wonder: isn't this the concern of the doctor not the patient? Isn't it the doctor's exclusive job to come up with the proper diagnosis and options for treatment?

Exactly. The standard doctor-patient model is to trust the doctor rather than leave it to the layman to make the discriminating judgments: the doctor is the expert, the patient, a more or less passive consumer whose main responsibility is to pass on relevant information about symptoms and response to treatment. Then if the doctor's magic doesn't work, either the patient returns to the clinic for new juju or cans the doc in favor of someone who can get the job done. The process repeats itself until the patient gets the right advice or is placed on life support and reduced to nodding and gagging.

I had long ago jumped ship on this relationship with doctors, and more generally, this orientation with the professional world. I was already a difficult person for most doctors and any other credentialed figures of authority interested in my health, savings, vote, or salvation. I was naturally suspicious of all plaques mounted on an office wall and most of all, anyone who punctuated a professional opinion with the phrase, "trust me."

Although I wasn't old enough to be a curmudgeon, I was sure I had the right stuff. Ask me to place my hand on the Bible, the Sutras, or the Upanishads and I will swear to God, Buddha, and Krishna that by far the best car I ever had was a used 1964 Barracuda with a bubble window and a push-button transmission. I am equally certain that personal computers waste more time than they save, and that cell phones mainly benefit people who frequently run out of gas on the freeway or are so insecure with family they need to provide regular reports that they are headed home from work, the grocery store, or the dog groomer.

I wasn't brought up by Communists under a toadstool, but there are socialists and other rose-colored apples in my family tree, and more than a few irreverent artists and poets, all of which probably account for my disengagement from the American mainstream. At an early age, I learned to explore on my own because of an encouraging mother with unbounded curiosity, and an incurious and absent Navy father.

By high school, I was a non-conformist with an identity anchored in football and journalism, and a love of the Navy which I expected to pursue at Annapolis. I might have actually become a midshipman except for the Vietnam War, which I saw as unjustified and based on deceit, particularly after the Gulf of Tonkin Resolution.

All this created a sore disappointment for my father, not only because he had hoped that I would go to the Academy, but because I was clearly questioning his long-held belief in America—right or wrong—and his certainty that an American President and his military commanders would never unnecessarily take the country to war. The rift between us only widened when I went east to attend Harvard in 1967.

College affected me in ways I couldn't imagine. Suddenly I was immersed in a world of ideas and falling under the influence of brilliant, iconoclastic teachers like James Watson, the molecular biologist of DNA fame; Howard Zinn, the Boston University historian; William Alfred, the classicist; James Thompson, the sinologist; Stanley Hoffman, the foreign policy expert; and Roger Revelle, the oceanographer. I learned to write succinctly, read with greater discrimination, and maybe most importantly, integrate and make connections between disparate ideas. It was a good time for that when the country was full of so many bright people willing to question and debate why we were in Vietnam, why civil rights were still being denied to so many, and how and why so many decisions in people's lives were dictated by large corporations exercising power through government, the media, and the marketplace.

During college years, I was affected by many books, but one above all others contributed to my world view: T.S. Kuhn's *Structure of Scientific Revolutions*. It demonstrated how whole bodies of scientific knowledge can be suppressed by gatekeepers at established institutions, in academia, by government, or the Church. It also illustrated how brilliant scientists dedicated to objectivity and dispassionate reason can be victimized by uninspected, self-serving biases.

The next major book to have such a profound effect came many years later. In the early 1980s my then-new friend, Madeleine, gave me a copy of Sheldon Kopp's *If You See the Buddha on the Side of the Road, Kill Him*. It sang harmony with T.S. Kuhn but in the realm of psychology and philosophy. In the best tradition of Buddhism, Kopp wrote, "The most important things that each man must learn no one else can teach him. Once he accepts this disappointment, he will be able to stop depending on the therapist, the guru who turns out to be just another struggling human being." I was sure this could be said of authority figures in most fields, be they scientists, public leaders, doctors, or critics.

So this was the mindset I brought to Cheswicke Hospital when my mom was struggling for her life in 1998. I had become a prove-it-to-me kind of person, a person more than taken by the state motto of Missouri—"the show-me" state. My mom's experience at Cheswicke Hospital only buttressed my skepticism about self-professed experts and complex systems. She might have died from her lymphoma, but the way she died and the timing of her death resulted from a medical system that was out of control.

I really had nothing personal against the doctors. In fact, I sympathized with most of them for living a demanding lifestyle that offered fewer and fewer rewards. Most were so overworked they had no home life, so burdened by exploding costs and paperwork that they didn't have enough time to spend with their patients. My own direct experience was that a diminishing number were able to find time to remain current in their own field, least of all, an allied one.

My friend Madeleine had several doctors as friends or clients, one of whom was a retired pediatrician named Maury, who left his practice prematurely because of the endless paperwork, squabbles with insurance companies, and skyrocketing costs. Madeleine frequently passed on Maury's observations about the state of the medical world.

Not long after my mother's death, Madeleine related to him my curmudgeon conclusion not to trust anyone invoking the phrase, "trust me." Maury apparently replied that there was an important corollary that I had missed—"Be especially suspicious if the phrase is uttered by a doctor." He was recently suffering from a botched eye operation.

His best recent assertion was that many of the finest doctors were giving up medicine to sell jewelry out of a briefcase. Supposedly, he had two close friends, old classmates from NYU medical school, who were now working the streets of Manhattan and doing quite well. Several of his old colleagues were still in practice but he suspected they were taking night classes in gemology.

I wasn't sure about Ralph Golan. I saw no sign of a bulging briefcase or jeweler's magnifying glass. Whatever his long-term scheme, I was confident of one thing—he was a sophisticated systems person. I had been a consulting ecologist for fifteen years and knew a bit about that. His book spoke my language—expressing relationships in terms of pathways, common denominators, triggers, linkages, threshold conditions, and interactions. When he answered my question in his office about inflammation in terms of levels and points of origin, I felt like a rhythm guitarist united with the right lead— Jimmy Hendrix on wheels.

His book contained a section on adrenal fatigue that caught my attention. "Everyone encounters stress in their lives. However, when the intensity and chronicity of stress surpasses a level beyond which an individual can cope, something is going to break down." The book contained a handy-dandy self-examination of life stressors. I took the test and my numbers blew out the scale. Besides the loss of my mom, I was trying to deal with the break-up of my business (an environmental institute), a family fight over my mom's estate, and discouraging rejections of my unpublished novels.

In another section labeled "The 10 Common Denominators of Disease" he sketched out an intricate relationship between stress, spiritual well-being, and immune function. Although most people are familiar with immune suppression and the problems of AIDS and chemotherapy, they are less aware that many immune system disorders are associated with an overactive response, which is the case with one hundred-some diseases.

One of the most important pathways by which stress affects health is through yeast infections. Besides its effects on respiration, liver, adrenals, thyroid, and kidneys, stress can prompt poor eating habits, which commonly lead to yeast overgrowth. A profusion of yeast, if unchecked, can erode the walls of the intestines, permitting yeast as well as other microbes to pass into the bloodstream.

The body's response to this is to sequester and kill the microbes once it discovers them in the blood. Most of us have seen the movie rendition of this—*The Fantastic Voyage*, in which T-cells and B-cells lead an orchestrated offensive against the evil invaders. In a body working properly, the good guys win and the immune system returns to normal, and hopefully the intestinal fissures are repaired that caused the initial release.

But for reasons that are not altogether clear, during some of the battles, the T-cells recapitulate the script of *Dr. Strangelove* and refuse to stand down, even when the threat is eliminated. The body goes into a kind of "DEFCON-1" mode, as a ghostly General Buck Turgidson continues to dispatch troops to defend his perimeter and B-52s to take care of the Rooskies. Unfortunately, there is no return to *fail-safe* and the T-cells trigger more and more inflammation, decimate healthy collagen, and generally overtax the body's energy stores.

This is one of the reasons that people with autoimmune diseases are frequently tired and exhausted. The syndrome is also self-reinforcing in that the more tired you get, and the more stressed you become, the easier it is for yeast to proliferate and for microbes to enter the blood stream.

I could relate to all of this. Especially after my mom's death, I was always tired and weak and even experienced yeast infections that I tried to control with Nystatin and friendly microbes like Bulgarus and Acidophilus.

What wasn't exactly clear from *Optimal Wellness* was how this syndrome manifested as psoriatic arthritis. The article that Ralph handed me in his office took off where the book ended. Although it didn't specifically address psoriatic arthritis, it suggested that many rheumatological diseases were caused by a very small l-class bacterium known as mycoplasma, a close relative of yeast and other fungi. Mycoplasma was parasitic. With no cell walls of its own, it could penetrate healthy collagen tissue and rely on host cells to meet its own metabolic needs.

The article stated that pioneering research on the subject was performed by Dr. Thomas McPherson Brown, a cohort of Albert Sabin, the noted polio doctor. From the late 1930s onward, Brown successfully treated thousands of patients using antibiotics. His protocol was now under study at Harvard's Beth Israel Hospital.

This was all I needed to send me on a Google search of Thomas Brown and his work. I quickly learned that he had written a book called *The Road Back* (subsequently reissued in expanded form as *The New Arthritis Breakthrough* by Henry Scammell and Thomas Brown, M. Evans, 1993). I ordered the book and read it in one sitting.

It told the dramatic story of Thomas Brown's life-long mission to understand and treat rheumatoid disorders and spun a compelling drama about a compassionate doctor doing everything in his power to help suffering patients. It provoked parallels to Oliver Sack's *Awakenings*, the works of R.D. Laing, and the story of Pierre and Marie Curie in trying to penetrate the mysteries of radium and radiation.

As a young doctor in the late 1930s, Brown worked as a researcher down the hall from Albert Sabin at the Rockefeller Institute. Sabin discovered a strange microbe in the brain tissue of a mouse, cultured it, and identified it as mycoplasma. He subsequently injected it into another mouse, which soon contracted rheumatoid arthritis. Almost simultaneously, Brown succeeded in isolating mycoplasma in the joint fluid of a human. This was the first powerful indication that mycoplasma might cause rheumatoid arthritis and related immune diseases.

Brown went on to develop a treatment that involved low-dose, long-term use of antibiotics, devised to apply relentless pressure on the microbe and eventually eradicate it. The regimen was premised on the fact that mycoplasma had developed an especially effective strategy of protecting itself from antibodies, utilizing the host cell's ability to encase and protect itself behind a lipid screen.

In Dire Straits

According to Brown, the same basic mechanics were involved in rheumatoid arthritis, psoriatic arthritis, scleroderma, Reiter's, Reynaud's syndrome, ankylosing spondylitis, lupus, and many other rheumatoid illnesses. What remained unclear (and perhaps attributable to genetic predisposition) was that the infections and subsequent inflammation seemed to target slightly different connective tissue (e.g., skin, back joints, hands, and knees). Each disease was also defined by a somewhat different progression and sensitivity to treatment. In all cases, however, Brown was certain that the immune system wasn't going haywire but simply flailing away at a very crafty and robust invader that had come up with an ingenious defense strategy.

Little did Brown realize that his ideas would be strenuously opposed by mainstream medical organizations, including the American Rheumatism Association. In the late 1930s and early 1940s, the "infectious theory" seemed to take hold, but thereafter most rheumatologists gravitated to the view that the body was simply suffering from a command and control problem.

Some rheumatologists were willing to concede that infection might be an initial trigger, but steadfastly maintained that long after it was eliminated, the immune system remained on tilt. Their focus was to reduce pain and dampen T-cell activity. The strategy was essentially designed to manage the disease rather than get at any underlying causes.

During WWII, steroids gained popularity and after that, methotrexate. Unfortunately, these were often associated with major side effects, and patients who showed initial improvements were seldom able to sustain them. In recent years, designer immune-suppressing drugs had become even more popular.

Money and corporate power played an important role in the argument between the two schools (infection versus haywire immune system). The pharmaceutical companies were no small player because of their financial power. Their interest clearly lay with immune suppression and the increasingly expensive label drugs that would accomplish this. The market for this was large because so many people—estimated at fifty million—suffered from autoimmune diseases. On the other hand, the financial gain from treating rheumatoid disease with tetracycline-class antibiotics was minimal (less than one hundred dollars per month versus much more for immune suppressors).

The history of Brown's struggle with the medical establishment could have been a chapter in T.S. Kuhn's book. For nearly fifty years, Dr. Brown tried to secure the funding necessary to test his theories. At virtually every turn, he was opposed by mainstream doctors who sat on the major boards and controlled the purse-strings. Undaunted, he continued to help thousands of patients who were discouraged and failing from the ravages of the diseases and the conventional drugs used to treat them.

One of Brown's most notable successes involved a gorilla named Tomoka. Throughout the 1970s, Tomoka was one of the main draws at the National Zoo in Washington D.C., in large measure because he was the first gorilla in the US to be born in captivity. Unfortunately, in the mid 1970s he developed a wasting, crippling arthritis.

By 1981, officials had lost hope in his recovery and were about to put him down. Hearing of the situation, Dr. Brown asked if they would consent to let him treat Tomoka with antibiotics. They agreed and every two weeks for three years Tomoka received an antibiotic I.V. Eventually, he experienced a remarkable recovery, regaining strength and mobility.

As a result, word began to spread that Brown was neither a crank nor a charlatan. Despite this, it wasn't until later in the decade that significant funding was allocated to study the efficacy of his antibiotic protocol.

In late 1988, on the publication of *The Road Back*, Dr. Brown appeared on ABC's feature news program, *20/20*. (At the time Brown was shaky and weak from cancer that would take his life a year later.) Unexpectedly, the interview turned into an unbalanced cross-examination of his ideas based upon questions supplied by his adversaries. Despite this, the program only spurred more interest in the antibiotic therapy and *The Road Back*, which sold fifteen thousand copies in two weeks.

As I read the book, I was struck by the fact that Brown's discussion of mycoplasma infections so closely fit my own medical history. He mentioned that a pneumonia incident commonly preceded the first rheumatoid flare-up. The sequence was as follows: 1. a major stressful event, 2. onset of fatigue, 3. pneumonia, 4. ballooning joints, 5. related rheumatoid symptoms. This was exactly what I experienced beginning in 1999, and onward to the fall of 2000.

Brown only implied that yeast or digestive track

disorders might be a contributing cause, but I was pretty confident that this was the case. I knew that mycoplasma had been widely discovered in the gut. The question was how did it get into the bloodstream? Golan seemed to answer this: through leaky gut, the syndrome by which intestinal lining becomes inflamed (e.g., by diet or stress).

As soon as I finished the book, I reached for the phone to share my thoughts with Madeleine. She already knew that I was reading the book and had questions of her own, but I couldn't contain myself. "It fits so perfectly—remember my bout of pneumonia in Denmark?"

"Yes, and you also had a childhood history of asthma attacks."

"I'm beginning to wonder if those attacks weren't really pneumonia episodes."

"From mycoplasma?"

"Exactly."

"And so the idea here is that the stress after your mom's death might have triggered the disease?"

"That's what I'm thinking. Combination of stress and fatigue and lots of grief."

"I've got to look at this book."

I promised that I would pass it on but I wanted to mine it one more time for relevant information. I re-read it twice more and with the turning of each page could only shake my head at the uncanny fit between what Dr. Brown was describing and my own progressive symptoms. I was even more certain that my difficulties had mainly been ushered in by the grief that followed that terrible shipwreck at Cheswicke Hospital.

In Dire Straits

Chapter 3

Grief and Gothic Fence Building

From a Buddhist point of view, grief is a form of attachment and suffering. There are many kinds of attachment. These include ties to people, possessions, places, ideas, and anything else that might give us comfort, sense of security, or meaning. The grief that people are most familiar with is the despair that follows the loss of someone close.

According to Steven Levine, one of my chief authorities on the subject, this kind of loss commonly provokes feelings of isolation, separation, and a sense of being in peril from a universe we're not sure we can really trust. He likens these feelings to the rope burns left behind in a tug of war when someone dear to us has been ripped away.

My own grief seemed to fit this perfectly. The struggle had left me exhausted, off-balance, and empty. In losing my mom, Gigi, I lost much more than a parent. We were confidantes and co-conspirators in matters of spirit and artistic discovery. We talked frequently; we shared our best insights; we knew what beat in each other's heart. If you are lucky, you have that kind of relationship with one or two people over the course of your life.

The youngest in a poor family of six children, Gigi was marginally educated and middling in terms of intellect. But she had one gift that by any standard was exceptional: an impetuous imagination that bloomed like a field of sunflowers. Even in her seventies, she was a dynamo of quirky creativity, curiosity, and vitality, at any one time working on at least two or three new projects. Among these were painting in oils, doll-making, playing and singing Broadway show tunes on the piano, directing a community drama group, raising roses, attracting exotic hummingbirds with the perfect feeder, playing golf, fixing broken appliances, scoring priceless finds at garage sales, and offering a helping hand to anyone she thought was an underdog.

At least twice a week I would call her for a full report on her latest breakthrough in painting, which she would deliver with the exuberance of a school girl, unless, of course, I had distracted her from the act itself, in which case, she would soon put me on hold, promising a quick return. It wasn't uncommon for her to lose track of time and leave me hanging. On more than a few occasions she would call me back three hours later and open with the words, "Now what were you saying?"

I loved her for the fact that creating was so important that it might turn her into an absentminded nincompoop. This could easily cause her to neglect an overflowing tub, a pot roast turning into charcoal in the oven, or an iron burning a hole in a pair of pants. The creative imperative had to be followed, even it took the house down in a fire. Not only was this the way she lived her life, but what she encouraged me to do as well.

I wasn't the only family member prone to creative excess. My mom sometimes painted in tandem with my great uncle Sky, a formidable western artist, noted for his radiant skies and desolate badlands, who had a habit of cluttering his paintings with camouflaged coyotes, decaying sheds, gnarled snags, and hideous vultures.

When I was seventeen, she recruited me to stabilize a rickety fence on the bulkhead behind our house in Seattle, Washington. Inside the house, the two of them were trying to save Sky's latest overwrought composition, which looked like a Hieronymus Bosch on drugs.

Minute by minute, our own artwork was becoming more overwrought and cluttered with pointless supports. At one point my mom appeared and announced, "Finally, you seem to be on the right track."

"Right track?"

That's all it took. Immediately we began fitting the fence with outriggers suitable for the Kon-Tiki, flying buttresses suggestive of Notre Dame, and cross members vaguely reminiscent of the Bridge on the River Kwai.

She loved that fence and didn't care one bit that it would blow over in the slightest summer breeze. Truth be told, she cared more about the artistic statement than any utilitarian solution. Anything worth doing was worth doing with quirky eccentricity and elan.

So this was the kind of person I lost when she died—not simply a mom, but a free-spirited friend, not simply a friend but a co-conspirator in some extravagantly mischievous Dada. The rope burns were all the worse because she died so abruptly.

In December of 1998, I visited her just before leaving on a business trip to the East Coast and Washington D.C. She was in good cheer, although a bit more serious than usual. She also complained about a pain in her back that had been bothering her for many months. A few weeks later I received an emergency phone call in Princeton, New Jersey to return home immediately. Her doctors had discovered advanced lymphoma in her spine and said she was in imminent danger of full paralysis. By the time I arrived on the scene, she was already on toxic, mind-altering drugs. Six weeks later, she died of hospital pneumonia triggered by chemotherapy.

The days that followed her death are a blur. The morning after she expired, a meeting was held at the mortuary to decide on funeral arrangements. I vaguely remember a scene that involved family members racing through a series of critical decisions.

Apparently, a lovely white box was selected, priced proportionately to show our great love for her as well as a premium stone to mark the grave. Someone scribbled out a note that I was responsible for composing an obituary by 6 p.m. and, if I could manage, a five or six-word inscription for the marker. That was needed even sooner. I was hoping that the Buddha would stand in for me but he had keeled over in exhaustion after three days of sleepless trauma at the hospital. Apparently we moved on to decide the details of the funeral service, including the perfect minister to speed Gigi on her way to Christendom, the quality of paper in the memorial program, and the deluxe crackers and mints that would be available in the reception room.

Five days later, I was summoned from sleep by the ringing phone: time to get to the mortuary for the service, the gravesite for the burial, and then back home for the after-burial party. Apparently we were on an airtight train schedule that afforded no delay. A single minute sacrificed to reflection or tears and all the bodies, dead and alive that were supposed to be onboard, would be abandoned to some backwater bardo.

I had barely been installed in my seat at the mortuary chapel when a righteous young minister, full of fundamentalist zeal, rose to the pulpit and began shaming the congregation with a message that everyone was ticketed for equatorial heat if they didn't embrace Jesus as their personal Savior.

For a moment, I thought my mom might pop up from her coffin and declare, "Wait a minute. What's going on here? I don't buy any of this. Someone help me out of this pimp mobile they are calling a casket." Fortunately a few of my more rebellious cousins rose to de-evangelize the service by relating humorous, joy-filled moments with my mom. Most of them involved some kind of sin or unholy mischief. My mom was a notorious trickster with a raucous laugh. If she ever thought someone were getting too pompous, they were slated for serious lampooning.

When the post-service party mercifully ended, I was left alone in the silence of my mom's house. I stayed there for most of the next few weeks, wondering if she might still be hovering about. In *The Tibetan Book of Living and Dying*, Sogyal

Rinpoche, had suggested that souls frequently linger after death and during these periods, one can sometimes communicate with them. I was quite sure that if my mom did any lingering, it would be here, among her unfinished paintings, her chirping songbirds, and wildlife that frequently visited our backyard.

Sogyal had suggested a practice known as *phowa* to reach disembodied souls in their afterlife transition and help them transition to a higher state. For several days, I intermittently followed the meditative practices outlined in the book. The closest I came to a connection with my mom was finding her in several of my dreams. Unfortunately, the dreams contained no animated dialogue, certainly none of the gushing exuberance we shared before she died.

The book did offer some comfort, however. I discovered that Tibetans had a much different attitude toward death than in the West. Sogyal told the story of a senior Tibetan monk who couldn't restrain his tears over the death of his master. "Why are you crying?" asked a younger Buddhist brother, curious over such an emotional reaction that seemed to belie attachment. "Because I am sad," answered the grieving monk unrepentantly.

Sogyal Rinpoche described his own sadness over the death of his master, Jamyang Khyentse. "...losing Jamyang Khyentse was a loss so enormous that I still mourn it, so many years later. My entire childhood had been lived in the sunlight of his presence...His words, his teachings, the great peaceful radiance of his presence, his smile, all of these are indelible memories for me."

Quite often a Tibetan family and sometimes an entire community would gather for days after a person's death. The principal intent was to ease the person's passing, but the ritual also supported those in grief. There was no imperative for anyone to hold back their tears or to move on, and this seemed to ease the adjustment for those that grieved.

This was so different than anything I had ever witnessed in America. Too often it seems that people in the West expect the bereaved to bounce back quickly from a loss. One author commented that everyone is bound by the ninety-day rule: you have three months to return to your old self, or your friends have the right to consider you psychologically wounded and let you stew in your own juices.

This was reminiscent of the Jerry Seinfeld episode in which a fellow known to Jerry, Elaine, and Kramer, falls into a coma. The girlfriend of the poor guy immediately makes a play for Jerry. "Take me now," she demands across the motionless body of her friend. Jerry demures and she tries to cow him. "Are you a man? What kind of man would be afraid of someone in a coma? Take me. Take me now." Jerry backs away, then later queries Kramer regarding the etiquette for someone in a coma. Kramer replies that there is no etiquette— the person has twenty-four hours to pull out of it and if he doesn't, everything is up for grabs.

In the aftermath of the funeral, I was the man in the coma. Relatives began to appear at my mom's house, marking the paintings and memorabilia that they had designs on and carting off other property that they wanted. I was still too dazed to object, still occupied spinning imaginary stupa wheels that might speed my mom's passage through the spirit world.

I noticed that every so often I would be jolted out of reverie by a strange vibration. At first I figured it was simply my latest pang of *dukkha* (life friction), or perhaps the onset of a panic attack, only to discover that the inheriting relatives were jacking up my mom's house, placing it on wheels, and preparing to roll it to market. Cashing in the small estate was the highest imperative.

Madeleine helped me pull myself together and it dawned on me that I didn't need to go along with the rushed liquidation. The sale of the house could wait until fall. This would allow me to tend to my mom's garden. That was always important to her. She had been looking forward to the spring planting. Now, I would take care of that for her.

Planting and tending to the garden was a healing act. I sieved the dirt with my bare hands and attentively observed the hard work of the night crawlers and pollinators. With an artist's eye, I counted the segments of the worms and imprinted the drone of honeybees, whose song became a kind of mantra that allowed me to empty myself of anxiety.

With the seeds turning into sprouts in the garden, I turned more of my attention to reading and self-reflection, trying to address my own wounds. Madeleine made several offerings to my weekly stack of spiritual explorations. These included the works of Steven Levine, Ram Dass, and several Buddhist authors.

Levine wrote that when you love someone deeply, they enter into your heart. Their death may literally be disheartening, causing chest pain or shallow breathing and releasing a freshet of chaotic emotion. For more than a few people, this includes feelings of isolation, fear, and even panic or anger. I had felt almost all of this since the funeral.

A few months after the funeral, one of the family members found an old trunk in the attic that contained my mom's homemade cloth dolls. The relatives took what they wanted but left me with the prize doll we had always known as Buffy. She was the size of a small child and boasted a protruding belly, cherubic face, and mischievous smile. We had always considered her a troublemaker.

Madeleine read my delight and entered into fantasy with me about Buffy's escape from the trunk, her weakness for chocolate, and interest in learning to walk, sing, and perform. On Halloween of that first year (1998), Madeleine I devised costumes for all the dolls and our combined collection of teddy bears. I'm sure a psychologist would claim that we were rapidly regressing into infantile fantasy, but Buffy added joy and a playful dimension to our friendship.

Soon after Buffy's arrival, I discovered the Buddhist author, Pema Chodron, who talked about "bringing death into everyday life." The thrust of this was to free yourself from fear and to surrender to the prospect of death. In so doing, you would gain greater appreciation for meaningful relationships. This made perfect sense. So much of life in America was about deluding yourself that you would never grow old. Plastic surgery, implants, Botox, and Viagra would take care of that. Old age was something to be pitied.

I was already well into middle age and had no illusions about everlasting youth. On more than a few occasions, I felt that life was passing me by, but this hadn't flowered into full neurosis. So far I had resisted elaborate charades to mask my receding hairline and restrained myself from scheming on women half my age. Though I was rebelling at least once every two years for a free-form trip to Europe with a backpack, I hadn't yet signed on with Peter Fonda and Dennis Hopper to smoke weed and fly through the sinuous streets of Monaco on a Harley road hog.

Chodron suggested that suffering (and presumably middle-aged angst) could be reduced by renouncing desire and passion (sometimes referred to as the Second Kesha). I wasn't exactly sure what she considered passion. If it were simply craving, the kind associated with addiction or over-indulgence, I could see her point, but I couldn't quite agree if she included sensory passions—the kind that motivated exploration and discovery and the brushstrokes of creativity. I certainly wasn't ready to kill that to free myself from grief.

Even Lama Surya Das, another of my favorite writers, seemed to agree with Chodron about the perils of passion and sensory indulgence. He drew upon the Buddha's Diamond Sutra in advocating a "Teflon mind" that clings to nothing. Others also suggested that enthusiasm and exuberance were forms of desire that needed to be controlled.

I didn't doubt that this would remedy much suffering, but taking this to the extreme would surely result in a flat-line existence—certainly none of the joyful artistic exploration that gave my own life meaning. Was that the suggestion?

Jack Kornfield seemed to resolve my confusion by suggesting that emotion shouldn't be renounced but mediated by awareness. You didn't kill craving and sensory delight, you just brought awareness and mindfulness to them.

A second book by Steven Levine spoke to me like none other. In *Who Dies* he wrote that grief is often about loss of a mirror. The people that we love most are our mirrors. They are people who recognize and pay tribute to the person we are or want to be. Though I had several close friends, Gigi was unique in her creative exuberance—the quality that she supported in me and that sometimes I doubted when life became difficult.

She always amazed me that she could recover so quickly from something that would discourage others. Even after the funeral of a close friend, she would soon be working on a new painting or doll. She was possessed with the drive to create, no less than a more talented professional or even the greats like Michelangelo, Vermeer, and Van Gogh. She had imparted this drive to me as well, although I had to admit that I was more easily side-tracked and discouraged when faced with rejection. I guess that was a difference between us: my fences needed more support than hers. She was more accepting of the possibility that no one would appreciate something she was really proud of.

A story from Ram Dass's *How Can I Help?* leavened my spirits. He spoke of trying to comfort a couple whose daughter, Rachel, had been abducted and murdered. The parents were beside themselves with grief. Ram Dass wrote, "Rachel came through you to do her work on earth. Now she is free...."

It was a simple but comforting thought. It reminded me of the words of Sogyal regarding his master. In both cases, the dead person's work was about imparting something important to a loved one left behind. If anything, Gigi's gift to me was about finding freedom through creativity. Many people came to her for inspiration and creative boost but I was her closest confidante. We laughed together; we created mischief; we divined cockeyed and crazy schemes. This was a connection I was most grateful for.

Later that first year, I decided this was something that required celebration, if only I could figure out the right gesture. Unfortunately I just couldn't seem to come up with anything that really captured the spirit of our relationship.

In fall of 1998, I escaped for a month-long trip to Europe. After an extreme case of pneumonia in Denmark, it came to me in a twilight reflection that I should go to Venice. This would be the perfect homage to her spirit. Venice was the one place we had talked about seeing together—visiting the canals, indulging our love of Renaissance art, drawing and painting.

My stay in Venice turned out to be a voyage of personal discovery, full of much synchronicity, play, and art. Somehow I stumbled upon a quaint four-star hotel willing to offer me a special rate because of a last-minute cancellation. The hotel fronted on a scenic side canal filled with skiffs and other working boats owned by locals. I used the hotel as my base of operation for daily exploration, during which I filled a sketchbook with images of people as well as bridges and ornate buildings dating back to the Renaissance. This was just the kind of trip my mom would have loved.

A few weeks later, I caught a long-haul train from

Munich to Nantes and reached for my travel journal. Suddenly I was recapitulating my recent experiences and reflecting on the transformative power of travel. Out of this came *The Mindful Traveler*, a book that was as much about inner as outer exploration, about using travel to deepen self-understanding and discover higher self.

A few weeks after the book was published, I decided to contact Steven Levine in New Mexico to let him know how much his own writing had meant to me in my darkest days. It wasn't easy to locate his number, but I discovered it by process of elimination. (I presumed that he would be located somewhere near his well-known clinic.) I didn't talk to him personally, but left a grateful message on his answering machine.

Two days later, I got a heartful reply on my own answering machine. "My name is Steven Levine. I am not the Steven Levine who is doing all the wonderful work with the sick and dying, who has written with such insight about grief, but I wanted to let you know that I feel truly blessed to have the same name as someone so compassionate. I only hope that I can be of service the way he has been. I wish you the best with your book, which hopefully will vitalize the spirit of others."

It was the perfect grace note for *The Mindful Traveler*.

In Dire Straits

Chapter 4

Landing Flies on a Dime

Within days of finishing Dr. Brown's book, I visited *The Road Back* website which offered a bibliography on articles about the antibiotic protocol as well as a bulletin board on which patients posted questions and answers about the many subjects discussed in the book. I was soon headed for the University of Washington Medical School Library where I essentially took up residence for the next month, scouring anything relevant about rheumatoid diseases and antibiotic therapy.

The articles I tracked down included studies from the Netherlands, Israel, and the University of Nebraska. Results confirmed that antibiotic therapy was effective for both inflammation and joint mobility. The Nebraska study recorded a remission rate of forty percent after four years, while sixty-five percent of patients improved significantly. Positive but modest results were also recorded in the national study that Dr. Brown had fought so hard for—a double-blind investigation of the efficacy of minocycline in treating rheumatoid arthritis.

My follow-up appointment with Ralph Golan was more

of an oral study session than a conventional doctor's appointment. I verbalized my understanding of the therapy and why it worked, and he filled in the blanks with possible effects on T-cells and B-cells. At end, both of us seemed convinced that the protocol was worth trying, especially if I tested positive for the microbe. My one reservation—and I could tell that Ralph shared in this—was the time it might take for the protocol to work. If the lag were greater than six months I could lose the use of several joints. Two more fingers were already swollen and I was experiencing early morning dizziness and brain fog that sometimes lasted until noon.

Because of cost and insurance considerations, I decided to involve my regular primary care doctor in decisions about treatment. (He had provided the original referral for me to see a rheumatologist.) I only hoped he wouldn't be affronted by Ralph's involvement and my own assertiveness.

The next week I met with him to go over the draft plan. As it turned out, he was both supportive and curious, although I wasn't quite sure that he believed the treatment would work. As a licensed naturopath, his own predilection was in favor of an austere non-inflammatory diet, supplemented by herbs that would modulate the immune system. I thought this made sense as an adjunct and resolved to make his recommended changes which included more omega-3 oils, boswellia, curcumin, willow, sea mussel, and plant sterolins. He echoed Ralph's view that I should control yeast, especially if I began taking antibiotics. At end, he offered a prescription for blood tests recommended by Dr. Brown. These included a PCR DNA test, the most powerful test available for detecting mycoplasma.

While waiting for the results, I spent hour after hour soaking in the tub trying to reduce the swelling in my digits and usually with some book or journal article close at hand. Lying there turning into a prune, it dawned on me that since my appointment with Dr. Reece, I hadn't experienced a single panic attack or an outpouring of grief. All that I could imagine was that I had been so caught up in my health crisis that I had been distracted.

One of the books close at hand was Daniel Goleman's, *Vital Lies, Simple Truths*. It seemed to explain this. According to Goleman, "When anxiety crescendos into panic…its intensity captures thought and action." A powerful chemical cascade was triggered that included ACTH and endorphins. He added, "Tuning out threat is one way to short-circuit stress arousal."

This apparently is what I had done by focusing my attention on problem-solving. There were other ways to dampen the anxiety, including avoidance, denial, and even fantasy, but all of these were really a focus on symptoms and effects rather than underlying cause. I wasn't entirely opposed to that, however, if it would give me a bit of relief.

A book by the Dalai Lama expanded on how one might still inner-noise. In Buddhism, the practice of stilling anxiety was called "taming the wild elephant." Techniques included chanting and meditation. The Eight-Fold Path also recognized the importance of considering ego attachments that inflated perceived dangers and threats and provoked aggression, hate and other "afflictive emotions."

I was soon sharing this with Madeleine who had been

busy studying Dr. Brown's book. Her normally frizzy hair seemed a little more electric.

"I really liked the case studies," she declared, referring to the histories of Dr. Brown's patients, including Tomoka the gorilla. She especially liked the story of Curly, a likable, bald-headed angler who worked for an outdoor supply company. Until rheumatoid arthritis disabled him, he regularly toured the country at venues like Madison Square Garden, demonstrating an ability to land a fly on a dime at one hundred feet. By the time he found his way to Dr. Brown, he was confined to a wheelchair, discouraged, and clinging to a dwindling ability to exercise.

He was immediately drawn to Brown, who possessed a quiet and compassionate manner. Like most severe victims of rheumatoid diseases, Curly was accustomed to glum doctors offering little hope of improvement. Dr. Brown was upbeat and positive, assuring Curly that he would improve and be able to return to what he loved.

The young doctors that Dr. Brown was training were already affected by the prevailing pessimism among rheumatologists and Dr. Brown felt they needed an object lesson. With the other doctors present, he asked Curly if he would consider remaining in bed for two weeks: it was important not to exercise or take other medications, otherwise someone might claim that this accounted for any improvements.

Curly offered a meek protest, "Good God, if I don't have some kind of activity, I'll just fall apart."

Dr. Brown assured him that he wouldn't. In fact, in two

weeks he would be back on his feet. Somewhat apprehensively Curly agreed.

Two weeks later, Dr. Brown returned with several young doctors. By then Curly was restive, irritable, and anxious to get out of bed. As Dr. Brown disconnected the IV, he asked Curly if he had taken any drugs or exercised.

No he hadn't.

"When you were admitted, would you have been able to walk to the nurses' station?"

Curly's exasperation bubbled to the surface. "No, and by God, I don't think there is any chance at all that I can do it now, either. I came here in a wheelchair because I couldn't walk in the first place, and I've been lying here flat on my back ever since, going to seed."

Dr. Brown invited Curly to get up. After a moment's hesitation he stood up, then placing one foot ahead of the other, unsteadily made his way forward toward the nurse's station. He hadn't walked like this in ages. No one was more surprised than Curly himself. It was the first important demonstration to doctors of a younger generation that the therapy actually worked.

Other stories chronicled amazing turnarounds—reversals of lupus, scleroderma, psoriatic arthritis, juvenile rheumatoid arthritis, and related diseases. Kim Lofts from Albany, Australia, was diagnosed with crippling arthritis that prevented him from working and playing the guitar. Two years later, he was back to normal, working on an oil-drilling platform in the South China Sea and playing music again.

Lorri Fillenwarth, age twenty-seven, of Indianapolis

deferred to rheumatologists to control her own aggressive joint inflammation. They put her on cortisone, plaquenil, gold salts, and methotrexate that not only didn't work, but ushered in constant nausea, damaged her liver, and provoked early menopause. Finally, she had had enough and started the antibiotic protocol. In time, it stopped the disease progression, stemmed an overwhelming exhaustion, delivered her from a wheelchair, and allowed her to take walks without pain, climb stairs, and work in her yard and garden.

Madeleine surprised me by declaring, "You know, I think it's the perfect disease for someone like you."

"What exactly does that mean?" I chuckled.

"It's a compound systems problem with lots of unknowns, plus the symbolism is pretty interesting—all this business about camouflage and hidden microbes."

"I'm not sure it's my kind of pain. Then, too, I was hoping to take a few more trips to Europe. I suppose I could write a new book, entitled, *The Mindful Wheelchair Traveler*."

"Yes. There you go."

Madeleine always had a strange slant on what most people considered catastrophes. She had first introduced me to the works of Henry Miller and we often compared notes on his many books. Madeleine's ideas were similar to Miller's. She believed in rosy crucifixion—a title of Miller's trilogy—the notion that if you are on the right path, you are bound to go through a testing ordeal, a crucifixion of sorts, that offers lessons about higher self.

There seemed to be a fit between this and Buddhist philosophy, particularly the Tibetan notion that suffering was something to celebrate because it offered a broom to sweep away negative karma. The idea here was that suffering could sensitize you to longstanding attachments, increase your empathy toward others, and provoke greater compassion.

Sogyal Rinpoche often spoke of the illusions about security and fixity. Severe illness pricked that illusion. Especially in the West, we convince ourselves that we can eliminate all vulnerability. We armor and insulate ourselves with insurance, retirement plans, and support networks, but uncertainty and flux are unavoidable and eventually something penetrates our defenses. In the *Tibetan Book of Living and Dying*, he had written, "This constant uncertainty may make everything seem bleak and almost hopeless; but if you look more deeply at it, you will see that its very nature creates gaps, spaces in which profound chances and opportunities for transformation are continuously flowering—if, that is, they can be seen and seized."

The image of the flowering lotus is central to Buddhist philosophy. The lotus reflects the potential for renewal through an awakened spirit. The plant actually germinates in the muck at the bottom of a stream, pond, or bog, and sends its stems upward through the water column toward the sun. At the surface, it transforms into a radiant flower, red, pink yellow, or white. It is hard to imagine that something so beautiful could arise from such humble origins.

My primary care doctor left a message on my phone that my test results were back and that I should come in to review them. He left no hint as to what they indicated and was equally hooded when I arrived and took a seat across from him. As I expected, my sedimentation rate was elevated, which fit with the inflammation I was experiencing. He paged through the mycoplasma tests results and shrugged—"No hits."

I was at a loss. I was so sure of at least one positive result. "What about the mycoplasma pneumonia test? That was the one the book talked about most." He paged back through the results again. It was listed on the last page. I caught it even before he did.

"Positive," I declared.

His eyebrows arched with surprise.

"It had to be there," I declared. "The symptoms were too perfect." For a brief moment, I basked in the vanity of believing that I, too, had the ability to land a fly on a dime at one hundred feet.

Chapter 5

Cowgirl Angels

My primary care doctor wrote out a prescription and I started on minocycline the following week. Because of all that Dr. Brown had said, I knew that I shouldn't expect the kind of turnaround experienced by Curly Knowlton. The microbes were stealthy and quite often it took a year or more to see a change. I had also steeled myself for a Herxheimer reaction, the flu-like symptoms that usually occur soon after treatment starts. These are usually taken as a sign that the antibiotics are killing mycoplasma.

I was slightly surprised by no herx and increased the dosage to the highest recommended level. Still, there was no reaction. I wouldn't be discouraged. This wasn't an uncommon occurrence. Then too, my disease was psoriatic not rheumatoid arthritis, so reactions might be different.

What I did notice was an increase in morning dizziness that affected thinking, writing, and conversation. Dizziness had been mentioned as a possible side effect of the drug, but something that usually abated. The worst part of the dizziness was that it made me very irritable and difficult to be around.

Buffy and my bears usually ran for cover and stayed there until receiving an all-clear sign from the Buddha.

Of my several close friends, Madeleine was most affected by this. Our weekend get-togethers had always been rich with conversation about books and current events. Now I struggled to maintain attention and almost always got lost on a digression. If she spoke too fast, I had to slow her down. If one of her sentences wasn't perfectly clear, I was left behind trying to unpuzzle the ambiguity. She seemed to be revolving at 78 RPMs and I was stuck on slow-play. It was exasperating, and on more than a few occasions I lashed out at her, which only caused us both to recoil in glum silence.

We both thought that the dizziness might pass, but after another month there was no relief. At a loss, I reviewed the protocol and decided to switch to doxycycline, an alternative antibiotic occasionally used by Dr. Brown when patients had trouble tolerating minocycline. It was considered somewhat less effective.

Immediately, I noticed a slight improvement in the disorientation, but the doxycycline caused stomach and intestinal problems that made sleep difficult and killed my appetite. I seemed to be caught on the horns of a dilemma— stomach irritability or brain fog. I changed dosage and experimented with ways to coat my stomach, but couldn't find a satisfactory solution. After a month, I decided to switch back to the minocycline. This time the dizziness was less severe, but I still wasn't fully present and able to think clearly before noon.

Good friend that she is, Madeleine was willing to forbear

through this difficult period, slough off my snapping comments, and offer ideas for treating symptoms. I was increasingly concerned about the swelling of my feet because this affected my mobility. Occasionally, I had taken either aspirin or willow, but now was resorting to NSAIDs (non-steroidal anti-inflammatory drugs). Some of these were quite strong but they only proved to be marginally effective, at least at the low doses I was willing to take. Just to get through the crisis, I decided to return to Dr. Reece for prednisone shots.

I hadn't seen him since my initial appointment. Not much had changed in his office. The same lost souls seemed to be waiting to see him and I wondered whether they had ever left the clinic. The doctor, himself, was just as cheerless and fatigued. While administering the shots, he asked how the methotrexate had been working out for me. I replied that I was taking minocycline instead.

He couldn't hide his skepticism and disapproval. He had "heard something" about antibiotic therapy, but doubted that it would work. I rattled off some of the statistics from one of the studies. He only replied that I might want to consider the new drug Enbrel, which he had played a role in developing and testing. He handed me a flyer.

"There is currently a waiting list, so the drug is rationed to those who have been on methotrexate for a year."

"That sounds like a pretty bad bargain." I answered. What I really wanted to say was that I had reviewed the biostatistics and still thought that minocycline was still more effective and less risky, but I could tell that he had neither the time nor inclination to discuss the matter with a patient. This was a Type I authority doctor, the diametrical opposite of Ralph Golan.

The prednisone caused my swelling to subside for a few days, but then, as I feared, it returned with the power of a sledgehammer. I headed for the tub and after several weeks of soaking realized a moderate improvement.

The Road Back homepage offered a lifeline during this difficult period. The bulletin board made it possible to compare notes with others experiencing similar problems. They frequently spoke of their own appointments with disbelieving, unsupportive rheumatologists. Quite often the doctors would offer bleak warnings of what would happen to you if you refused methotrexate and chose an antibiotic protocol. It was as if the patients were taking snake oil.

The irony was that they seldom seemed to apply to the same standards of proof to their own remedies that they demanded of Dr. Brown. They didn't even have an explanation as to why immune cells would suddenly begin attacking healthy tissue. About all they could offer up was a vague black-box theory that genetics were involved. Didn't it seem much simpler and even a direct application of Occam's Razor to assume that an immune system had actually been revved up by infection, albeit a very small microbe-like mycoplasma that everyone knew was difficult to tag because of its lack of cell walls? Moreover, it was well established from the late 1930s that you could inject joints with bacteria and trigger arthritis.

Even shakier were the alleged efficacy and safety of conventional therapy—DMARDs (disease modifying arthritis drugs). These included gold salts, methotrexate, and steroids.

Dr. Brown hated gold. It masked symptoms and its effects included lung and kidney damage. The effects and side effects of methotrexate depended on dose and regimen. One prominent authority, David Trentham, M.D., of Beth Israel Hospital, was quick to note that at best, it only worked for two to three years.

Dr. Brown attributed much of the dismissal of antibiotics to a bias in medical school training. Most rheumatologists new very little about their use in treating autoimmune diseases. You really had to dig to find medical journals that discussed antibiotic therapy.

I was sure that the bias, especially in recent years, reflected the power of the drug companies. The largest pharmaceuticals devoted millions to new lines of immune-suppressing drugs. The literature in every rheumatology office gave evidence of the impressive ad campaign masked as public information.

The doctors themselves benefited in ways that they didn't often admit, enjoying subsidies for travel to attend lavish conferences and receiving lucrative stipends to be listed as members of an oversight committee that supposedly had reviewed a new and expensive designer drug.

The Arthritis Foundation itself, the main association devoted to the treatment of arthritic diseases, was funded by large drug companies and devoted much of its reporting to the discussion of the new drugs. Antibiotics were hardly ever mentioned.

The Road Back protocol suggested that slow-responders could jump-start their therapy by taking clindamycin IVs. This was the treatment that had brought Curly Knowlton to his feet. It seemed time for me to try them as well.

My primary-care doctor said he was willing to administer the IVs, but because he was a naturopath, needed oversight by an M.D. (an injunction under Washington State law). This proved to be less of a problem than I expected and within a few days I was at the clinic receiving an IV drip of clindamycin.

The procedure went off without a hitch for the first few days, but because no one was working on the weekend, I had to find another doctor or nurse to administer the cocktail for the last two days.

I thought I had located an available doctor and made a late Friday visit to his clinic to confirm the appointment, only to learn that complications had arisen and he couldn't help. Chagrined that it was now too late to find a stand-in, I meandered toward the door. I had just reached for the handle when a whisper stopped me in my tracks.

"I think I know someone who can help you," came the voice behind me. A lady handed me a scrap of paper and slipped away.

I figured I had nothing to lose and called the number. Two phone calls later I reached a freelance, practical nurse named Sarah, who assured me that she was the person I was looking for. I simply had to show up at her house over the weekend with my medication and she would handle the rest. Naturally I should be prepared to pay in cash.

She lived in a modest neighborhood just south of Seattle where at least half the houses had a mobile home parked in the driveway. I was on my way to the front door when a pickup truck pulled into the driveway and a shapely forty-year-old woman emerged, wearing skin-tight jeans, a form-fitting riding jacket, a low-cut tank top, and turquoise costume jewelry.

"I hope you haven't been waiting long," she declared with a Texas twang.

"No problem whatsoever."

She was not only attractive but very friendly and down to earth. She led me toward the house with a confident but unabashed stride—a model or dancer but without affectation.

"I had to make a home visit. Weekends can be pretty hectic," she declared buoyantly.

"Somebody else who needed an IV?"

"People got to get their meds," she smiled, making fleeting eye contact.

She unlocked the front door and beckoned me to follow. At once I was staring at one of the largest collections of Thomas Kinkade paintings I had ever seen. She broke my gaze and directed me toward a nook in the living room adorned with family photos.

I was staring at a picture of Sarah seated on a thoroughbred, when she declared, "Been riding since I was a little girl—dressage, jumpers, even used to exercise thoroughbreds before I became an LPN."

I nodded. It explained her tight athletic body. She removed her jacket and was now showing a bare mid-drift. Showing no discretion whatsoever, I took a deep draw from the well.

"Let's take a look at your veins," she declared, obviously

aware of my interest. I held out my arms and she bent from the waist revealing ample cleavage contained in a frilly black bra.

"Piece a cake," she shot back with a smile. I handed her the instructions for preparing my medication and she retired to a back room. It suddenly occurred to me that I was entrusting my veins to someone I didn't really know.

She said she was an LPN, not an RN. Did I want an LPN mixing my meds and inserting a catheter into my arm? If the needle or catheter weren't sanitary, I could be risking serious problems. On the other hand, she did seem pretty confident. Then, too, she had a frighteningly beautiful body. Even the Buddha noticed that.

I was trying to reconcile the two divergent philosophies about emergency medical treatment, one based on sensuality, the other on credentials, when she reemerged. In one fluid motion, she wheeled a lamppost next to my chair with her right foot, dropped an IV bag over the top with her left hand, and started to bleed the bag with her right. It was an impressive show of dexterity. That was always the quality you looked for in a good exercise rider. I knew a bit about race riding from junkets to the local racetrack.

"You probably do this a lot," an escaping voice declared.

"More often than you can imagine."

She placed my arm on a tray and inspected it again while bending from the waist.

"Yup, no problem whatsoever." I was utterly confident that she was wearing Victoria's Secret—probably Victoria's Secret for cowgirls. Before I could take a deep breath, my bicep was in a lasso, and the catheter was in my vein. She tapped the line confidently, and I could see that I was drawing clindamycin. This woman was a pro.

"Just relax," she smiled reassuringly. "In ten minutes you'll be a new man."

"I think I am already," I grinned narcotically.

While the antibiotic seeped into my bloodstream, I gave her a quick explanation of the theory behind the therapy. She seemed to want more and I filled her in while a more sensual conversation was engaged with half glances and inviting gestures.

"All done now," she declared suddenly. I was glad that at least one of us was paying attention. "That worked out pretty well, don't you think?"

"Maybe we should do it again."

"That's an idea," she grinned. "Only slower."

I sighed and she retired with the paraphernalia to another room. She met me at the door where I handed her one hundred dollars plus a fifty-dollar tip. She dropped it down her bra, then reaching for the door declared, "Give me a call any time you need some serious care."

"I'll be praying for a setback."

In Dire Straits

Chapter 6

Mycoplasma and September 11

The hardest part of those first six months was adjusting to the unpredictability of the disease. The IVs didn't immediately help, but a month later I improved for no apparent reason. A few weeks after that, I crashed again. Each setback provoked a certainty that the disease was spiraling out of control, and each improvement triggered an optimism that I was headed for recovery.

Madeleine was the only one of my friends who was really aware of the roller coaster I was on. Others knew that I was struggling, but couldn't quite believe that my problems, if they were real, could be caused by any form of arthritis. Many of them had less inflammatory osteoarthritis or some kind of joint discomfort, but never let it get in the way of work or play.

From my reading and web browsing, I discovered that this was a common reaction. Most people imagine that rheumatoid disease is simply a joint problem and usually a slow and progressive one that can be handled with mild anti-inflammatory drugs. The idea that your joints could be under aggressive attack doesn't seem to register. There is even less awareness of the systemic complications often associated with the diseases—extreme fatigue, sleep problems, muscle aches and strains, sprains and tears of connective tissue, dizziness, adrenal overload, vision problems, irritable bowels, skin problems, depression, and even coronary disease.

I was chagrined to discover that mycoplasma pneumonia was often one of the more aggressive microbes. But then again, I already suspected that my problems were a little more severe than most rheumatoid and psoriatic cases. Madeleine had reached the same conclusion. The one consolation was that antibiotics often seemed to work more quickly on aggressive strains than milder ones. I just hoped I would soon begin to respond.

Over time, I quit talking about my problems to all but my closest friends. If a casual acquaintance asked how I was doing, I said fine and then hoped they didn't notice the condition of my hands or my slight limp. If they did, I would usually slough it off and divert discussion to another topic. On occasion, I would run into someone practicing the same basic camouflage and we would share an instant recognition. Most people didn't want to be singled out for pity or uncomfortable questioning.

I was lucky that I didn't have to face the difficulties of working in an office. Work poses a difficult problem for people with severe rheumatoid diseases. If you continue to work, you certainly want your boss and co-workers to believe that you can handle your responsibilities. Admitting a problem could easily ticket you for reassignment, demotion, or even unemployment. Because of this, joint problems are often disguised as injuries from accidents or sports, rather than something chronic that might worsen.

The cover-up can be as elaborate as the schemes of a closet alcoholic. At meetings seated around a conference table, people will hide their swollen hands beneath a table or find ways to screen them from direct view. Because fatigue is a constant problem, employees will find ways to rest or nap. "Just resting my eyes," will be the claim of the person conked out at their desk. Then there will be the afternoon checkouts to work at home, except that you streak for the tub or bed rather than to a computer.

For the moment, I had enough savings so that I didn't have to work at a regular job, but I needed the income from the sale of my books and this required promotion. I normally enjoyed book signings and the opportunity to speak to groups but I was increasingly concerned about my credibility. Who, after all, was going to take a travel author very seriously who wasn't traveling, especially if they noticed him limping? Truth be told, my most ambitious recent travel consisted of getting from my bed to my orthotic shoes and then to my car, if I could find it (not always easy to remember where it was parked if I were dizzy). Then the ordeal really began of reaching the pharmacy or grocery and getting back home before complete exhaustion. This wasn't exactly *Video Night in Kathmandu* or *Riding the Iron Rooster*, two of my favorite travel adventures, written about by Pico Iyer and Paul Theroux.

What really piqued my anxiety was giving a talk when I was dizzy, my usual condition until early afternoon. In this condition, I would often forget what I was saying and experience brain lock in trying to retrieve the most obvious information: "Yes, a few years ago I was in....you know, that Renaissance city in eastern Italy known for the canals... not Florence but...." I prayed that the Buddha would deliver me from my embarrassment and he usually did, but he always made me sweat.

To prevent embarrassment and debacle, I tried to schedule presentations for the evening, but this wasn't always possible. When I had to speak at an early hour, I put on a good façade and tried to keep it simple. Nevertheless, I'm sure that much of the time I came off as a drunken sea captain trying to negotiate the Golden Gate during a killer fog.

To forestall shipwrecks, I spent much time preparing. The night before an event, I would make elaborate notes and test myself with questions. In reviewing the book, it almost seemed that it had been written by someone else. So much of the message was about trusting your resourcefulness and learning to improvise while on the road, but I wasn't even getting to the road. In my current state, I couldn't possibly tote around a backpack. On any given morning, my first worry upon awakening was that a yawn or stretch would strain my neck and turn me into a bed-ridden jellyfish.

If I couldn't travel I could still find identity in being an occasional writer. This posed at least two problems. First, it was difficult to write without much recall, and then, when I tried to use a keyboard, my hands often swelled up. It was particularly difficult to use a mouse. I devised a number of fixes to alleviate pressure, including hand and wrist supports as well as compression wraps. I even learned to use a mouse left-handed. Sometimes the fixes worked; other times I had to be content reading and trying to write in longhand, which itself was a struggle.

The one great tonic for my spirit was that I was getting nibbles on an unpublished novel. Chris Merritt, a valued friend from Wisconsin, had agreed to represent me and together we managed to interest both a New York publisher and a major executive with DreamWorks. My heart soared. I really needed a shot of confidence for my flagging morale.

Unfortunately, the prompt decision that we both hoped for didn't materialize. For months on end we simply waited: waited for DreamWorks, waited for the publisher. I tried to be philosophical about it. Impatience was probably something I needed to work on, particularly as it related to my own slow healing. Maybe this was what all my European train travel was really preparation for—patience in dealing with delay and obstruction. If I could bear diversions of Italian trains and the frustrations of finding an affordable room in Paris, perhaps I could handle this.

In late summer of 2001, I was beginning to lose hope that I could avoid an operation on my hands. I hadn't been responding very well to occupational therapy and was pretty sure that at least one finger needed joint fusion. A basic problem was that from week to week, inflammation would rise and fall and prevent aggressive therapy to regain my range of joint motion. This also made me wonder whether surgery even made sense until the inflammation subsided. I didn't want to be wheeled in for one surgery and discover that I might as well have waited another month for an operation that included a second joint. A further uncertainty was whether the surgery itself might spread the inflammation to my larger joints.

I decided to see a surgeon at the University of Washington, widely considered one of best in the Seattle area. Hopefully he would know something about inflammation control and be familiar with the kind of dynamic problem I was dealing with. The appointment took over a month to schedule.

I thought I had carefully prepared for it but immediately realized that our interests were different. I was trying to deal with a moving train and he was only interested in stationary ones. As I aired my concerns about my inflammation, he only focused on my X-rays. In his view, the only important issue was the condition of my fingers and hands in the moment, not down the road. Any subsequent problem would have to be handled then. After a quick scan, he imperiously recommended surgery on two finger joints.

I pressed him further on possible repercussions and he grew short-tempered. "I'm a surgeon, not a rheumatologist. I can tell you that this one joint is completely trashed, hopeless; the other is marginal and the inflamed ones will be gone if you don't stop your disease, but again, anything you might do in this regard is beyond my expertise and concern."

I tried to elicit options other than surgery for the "non-trashed" joints and was interrupted by his ringing cell phone. He excused himself to take the call, and left me alone to stare at my sore hands. I had no idea whether he would be returning. I glanced up at the clock. He had given me five minutes of his time and a pretty clear choice: either get on board or forget it. Suddenly all my frustration erupted. No way I was going to be treated like this. I gathered my clothes and X-rays and strode past the doctor and his assistants who were talking casually.

"Will we be scheduling a surgery for you, Mr. Currie?" came the surprised voice of the doctor's nurse. I took all my self-control not to tell her what she could do with her scheduling.

In fall of 2001, I reached my limit in waiting for the antibiotics to kick in. I promptly made reservations to visit David Trentham, the Boston rheumatologist, whom most people considered the leading authority on the antibiotic protocol. Trentham was the principal investigator in the double-blind study that Dr. Brown had fought so long for.

As I prepared for my trip, the first significant travel in nearly three years, I reflected on the fact that I wasn't exactly embracing the credo I had been promoting with my book. It wasn't so much that I wasn't traveling, but that my life seemed to be controlled by voices of limitation. In the book, I had ticked off a host of voices that keep people from growing, exploring, learning, and solving simple problems. These include the voices of financial ruin, disability, and limited resourcefulness.

In most cases, the voices exaggerated and distorted a less-than-dire limitation. In the last several months, I had given ear to most of them. Even when I was generally showing equanimity and mindfulness, a minor bump in the road would throw me off balance, and then the voices would begin chirping, "You can't do this; you'll get in trouble if you do

71

that." It was a wonder that Buddha hadn't split the scene entirely. In traveling to Boston, I would try to be more positive, heroic, and outgoing. Otherwise it was time to go shopping for reverse earplugs that would mute the messages from my neurotic brain.

Then, the Trade Towers and Pentagon were struck by the terrorists. Suddenly, my own attention, like that of other Americans, shifted away from my own problems to the drama playing out in New York, Pennsylvania, and Washington. Public shock soon gave way to the uplifting images of prayer vigils and rallies, not only in America but Europe, Asia, and the other continents. It seemed that most of the world was coming together and extending their compassion to America and the families that were suffering.

On September 12, the United Nations Security Council passed a resolution condemning the terrorists and those aiding them. German Chancellor Gerhard Schroeder immediately offered an expression of unconditional German solidarity with America. *Le Monde*, the Paris daily, ran a headline that read "Nous sommes tous Américain (We're all Americans)." It was a rare moment of international brotherhood that seemed to promise cooperation and collective effort to eradicate terrorism and its causes.

As the media focused on Manhattan with twenty-four-hour TV coverage, it was unclear how the country would respond once the shock abated. In some sense, I was reminded of my own imbalance after the diagnosis by Dr. Reece. The temptation was to push the panic button. A poll in the *New York Times*, suggested that over seventy percent of Americans didn't feel retaliation was a good idea until we knew exactly who was responsible. I was surprised by the forbearance.

It was short-lived, stirred in no small way by the media and extreme columnists. The networks began displaying backdrops of waving American flags and the smoking trade towers. Simultaneously a chorus of right-wingers demanded immediate military action.

The cable TV commentator Ann Coulter quickly spoke out for an American invasion of countries that had harbored the hijackers. Their leaders should be killed and their people converted to Christianity. William Bennett and writers for the *New Republic* and *The Weekly Standard* threatened to brand George Bush as a wimp if he dithered in attacking Iraq. Jerry Falwell and Pat Robertson even suggested that gays and lesbians were somehow responsible for 9/11.

Within weeks, George W. Bush rallied the masses to a new crusade with the words, "You are either with us or you are with the terrorists."

The parallels were irresistible between the problems I had gone through with my immune system and what the country now seemed to be experiencing. A sneaky microbe had ghosted in under the radar, delivered a telling blow, and left panic in its wake. The immune system was now roused and ready to rock and roll. Parasites that they were, the bad guys seemed to be hiding among good freedom-loving folk and spreading more terror. That was going to end soon enough. Special forces would take care of 'em, killer T-cells and such. Only problem was that some friendly cells might be wasted in the process. Unfortunate but necessary. Call it collateral damage.

Any hope for a discriminating response seemed to wane with the discovery of anthrax in Florida and soon thereafter in New York. This coincided with the first bombings in Afghanistan, which in turn provoked widespread worry that Al Qaeda would re-retaliate with widespread bio-terrorism.

Within weeks, letters containing mysterious white substances appeared across the country. False alerts were rampant. The deadly Islamic mycoplasma now seemed to be fighting back. In three weeks the FBI responded to over 2,300 alarms at locations as diverse as LAX, Cape Canaveral, and the offices of Planned Parenthood. This prompted more fright and a run on ciprofloxacin, doxycycline, and gas masks. Borrowing from the practice of Israelis, Americans began turning their homes into plasticized bubbles to keep out the dreaded germs.

In the midst of the anthrax scare, I found myself checking my own supply of doxycycline. I still had plenty available since switching to minocycline. I passed the word on to Madeleine and told her that she and Buffy were covered in case the germ bomb hit. She answered that since I was probably protected from anthrax because of all the antibiotics in my system, I should do my patriotic duty by volunteering to check suspicious parcels for the post office.

Like so many other Americans, I was becoming a news junkie. I was also paying attention to the marginal print-stories and letters to the editor that seemed particularly revealing. In early October, several thoughtful letters appeared in the *New York Times*. Ron Lowe from Nevada City, California, wrote,

"Since Sept. 11, waves of fear have rocked the United States, and the false sense of safety and security has been shattered. There is an answer; there is a choice. Feed into fear, or call up some courage." I needed to tape this message to my bottle of minocycline.

On October 9, Pete Newman of Brooklyn wrote, "...To acknowledge that we or our loved ones could be facing imminent death as we relax in our homes or attend ball games is to accept the unacceptable truth that in the end we all die. It is difficult to admit that a heart attack, like an act of terror, can sneak up on us in the blink of an eye, that our lives could end suddenly. But we do exercise control over how we live. We must therefore live as honestly and courageously as we can while we can, never forgetting that we have an obligation to treat one another with decency because we might never get another chance."

Both letters resonated with the messages in Sheldon Kopp's books. Kopp had made the point that fear was about perceived vulnerability. Usually the perception was an exaggeration of the real threat. I recognized this from my own struggles with panic. The wild elephant always raged when you felt isolated and alone.

In *Raise Your Right Hand Against Fear*, Kopp had written about the danger of responding reflexively to fear. "Cautious consideration works better than impulsive action...Demonically driven, we may intentionally increase the likelihood of the jeopardy we fear." The message reflected Buddhist wisdom that anger and the impulse to payback were really forms of fear. I hoped that this wouldn't be exploited by politicians and military interventionists but the signs weren't very hopeful.

On October 11, a small article by Elaine Scotino caught my eye. She reported that a "tight group" of Pentagon officials and defense experts, referred to as the "Wolfowitz cabal," was arguing for a military operation against Iraq. They claimed a linkage between the events of September 11 and Saddam, and proposed invasion, takeover of Iraqi oil fields, and the replacement of Saddam by a friendly regime.

No mention was made of George Bush's position, but I was apprehensive. Iraq had been in the cross-hairs of Richard Perle, Paul Wolfowitz, and Bush's hawkish advisors since the end of the First Gulf War. Bush himself was known to have issues with Saddam over the assassination attempt on George, senior.

My misgivings only intensified on October 12, when Bush again reached for the twelve-gallon white hat and addressed the people of Afghanistan, "If you cough him up (Osama) and his people today...we'll reconsider what we are doing to your country." Then he offered a stream of garbled consciousness that suggested his view of himself, America, and the larger world. "The evil ones have sparked an interesting change in America, I think. I am amazed that there is such misunderstanding of what our country is about that people would hate us [sic]. I am like most Americans. I just can't believe [sic]. Because I know how good we are."

I recognized this kind of thinking. It was the same dizzy clarity I achieved in those early morning bookstore presentations. The one major difference, however, was that even when I was spinning upside down, I had no difficulty understanding why foreigners might have grievances with America. It was such a shame that George Bush knew so little about the world, had traveled so little internationally, and was so incurious.

I had no idea just how nervous people had become until I boarded a flight to Boston in late November and began observing behavior at the airport and on board the plane. It was an unspoken, mostly quiet fear that was ratcheted up further by news of more anthrax discoveries in Washington D.C. and New Jersey. Everywhere people seemed to be suspicious and ready to profile anyone who looked Middle Eastern, and all the worse if you possessed a Muslim-sounding name. If you were the Buddha it was time to consider a makeover and some late-night tutoring to rid yourself of that incriminating East Indian accent.

In Boston, I traveled across the river to Cambridge for a reading from *The Mindful Traveler* at Harvard Square. At the Harvard Coop, I briefly connected with a young Harvard undergraduate named Allison, representing *Let's Go*, the Harvard student-run travel organization. She spoke fearlessly of her resolve to keep traveling. (Already the airlines were hurting from mass cancellations.) For her it was indispensable to education. It expanded awareness of diversity; it exposed you to radically different points of view. It made you look at your own beliefs and values more critically.

I was surprised to find that Morris Berman, one of my favorite authors, was also giving a book presentation at the Harvard Coop just the night before my own. He had previously written two impressive books about philosophy and social history: *Coming to Our Senses* and *The Reenchantment of the World.* His new book, *The Twilight of American Culture,* asserted that a cultural shift was well underway in America and its earmarks were a dumbing-down of the education system, ascendance of an empty consumer culture, and the valuation of celebrity over and above achievement. This went hand in hand with a glorification of simple-mindedness that passed for wisdom and thoughtfulness.

I attended the talk and found it to be both provocative and powerful. Berman pulled no punches in linking September 11 to the themes in his book. He made a strong argument that the country had lost its ability to tell fact from fiction and was giving a free pass to its fear-mongering leaders.

The argument jogged my recall of the works of Ken Wilber, one of America's deepest thinkers. In his many books about spirituality and philosophy, he described a ladder of awareness whose lower rungs were dominated by primitive cravings and fear, ego, and narrow personal and tribal identities. Mindfulness was almost entirely lacking.

Societies, like people, got stuck at the lower levels. The ones caught up in nationalism, power struggles, and warfare seemed to have no mirror. They could only see the wrongs of others and the rightness of their own causes.

All of this reminded me of the Buddhist notion of deep listening. A runaway mind full of fear was incapable of picking up nuance. You had no ability to discriminate real threats from imagined ones; you tended to think in terms of simplistic dichotomies, friend and foe, members of the tribe and outsiders.

Buddhism also advocated meditation to make the leap to higher awareness, but this was never enough. You needed to confront your own attachments and how they distorted everything that entered your sensory field and converted them to threat and peril.

From my background in ecology, I knew that the ability to discriminate was critical to animal and species survival. The wildebeest at the waterhole depended on her ability to tell the log from the crocodile. If every log spooked her, she could never meet her other needs and would always be adrenalized and overly defensive.

Likewise, a society in a constant state of irrational panic was headed down the path of assured demise, reflexively squandering its limited resources and drawing down its reserves so that when it really was faced by mortal threat it was impotent and exhausted. Maybe that was what Osama Bin Laden was betting on.

I tailored my own talk to discuss ways that people could bring more mindfulness to their travels. This might include greater attention to security concerns but also the rise and ebb of your anxieties and how they governed your choices. I asked the audience to pay particular attention to voices of limitation and how they affected exploration and discovery.

I arrived for my appointment at David Trentham's office and was grateful to speak, at last, to someone who knew more than I about the antibiotic protocol. He examined my inflamed fingers and offered the opinion that only two looked irreversibly damaged. For these I would probably need joint fusion. The others might be saved if I could lessen inflammation. In order to maximize the effectiveness of the protocol, I should switch from generic minocycline to Minocin, which was significantly more potent. The switch had made all the difference for many patients. He wanted me to keep him posted on my progress after the first two months.

I was struck by the fact that he was so attentive. Of all the doctors I had seen since the onset of my disease, only he and Ralph had actually touched my inflamed joints and look closely at them. He also seemed to be listening to what I was saying about solving two problems at once: dealing with the inflammation as well as the underlying disease mechanism.

It was an encouraging appointment but for one exception: Trentham noted that psoriatic patients didn't respond as well to Dr. Brown's protocol as those with rheumatoid arthritis. Perhaps I would be an exception, but he couldn't say for sure.

Chapter 7

Mindful Travel at Home

While on the plane home, I decided that when I arrived in Seattle, I needed to make a diligent attempt to maintain the mindset of my trip. Even though the arthritis had presented many difficulties, I had found a way through them. Beyond that, I had actually found a way to transcend my personal worries, stay engaged in the larger world, and try to be of help to others struggling with their diseases. Now I needed to do more of that and maybe help alert people to the crazy, fear-based behavior that seemed to be overtaking the country.

Of course, I had made similar resolutions in the past—returning home energized and committed to keeping a travel mindset alive, and then had been overtaken by samsara, the struggles of daily life. I suppose I had certain advantages this time. Among other things, *The Mindful Traveler* had been published, which gave me some touchstones and reminders of ways to deal with bumps in the road and the ways egoic attachments unravel the best of intentions.

A few weeks after I returned to Seattle, I experienced acute swelling and inflammation of my hands and decided to seek out a hand specialist for possible surgery. Not wanting to repeat the experience at the University of Washington, I was resolved to be as cheery and solicitous in all my conversation with doctors.

My latest hand-surgeon candidate was the head doctor at the prestigious Formalin Clinic. For the first few minutes of my initial appointment I thought I was doing pretty well. I was generally cheerful and deferential, but did present the doctor with a list of priority questions. With no display of emotion, he scanned them quickly, offered brief opinions regarding the most important issues, and then declared, "I hope that takes care of your concerns. Now I must tell you that I can no longer see you as a patient or perform surgery on your hand."

I was dumbstruck.

"I only have ten minutes per patient and you have too many questions. I'm sure there would only be more after surgery."

"No," I protested meekly. "We've only taken ten minutes."

"Sorry, you'll have to find someone else. There is another surgeon at the university who might see you. My nurse can give you his name. Have a nice day."

I fell into glum reflection. I couldn't see that I had done anything wrong. I certainly hadn't babbled; I hadn't been insulting; I hadn't even questioned the doctor's authority, but my questions did suggest that I wasn't going to be a passive and undiscriminating drone. The issue, then, had to be liability. The doctors had to be viewing me as a trouble-maker who might sue if something went wrong.

Jim's Verboten Questions on Hand Surgery

1. Extent of irreversible damage to hands?
2. Progression/change since last seen?
3. Surgery—joint replacement for one or more fingers at a time?
4. Procedure—specifically what will be done? Tighten ligaments?
5. Material used and durability?
6. Nerve damage potential?
7. Continued use of doxycycline?
8. Post-surgery therapy?
9. Scheduling of operation—length of wait?

Not exactly sure where to turn, I wrote an overly long letter to Dr. Trentham, asking for advice, particularly in controlling my spiking inflammation. He wrote back a cryptic letter to see a senior Seattle rheumatologist named Wilske. Apparently Wilske was versed in the antibiotic protocol. This looked promising.

I immediately called Wilske's office and was soon speaking to his assistant, relating the recommendation from Dr. Trentham. She assured me that Wilske was the right doctor and "conversant in the full range of protocols for treating psoriatic arthritis." I made the earliest possible appointment—a month away. I just hoped my hands wouldn't be permanently damaged while I waited.

A month later I was seated in Wilske's office. He was congenial and kindly, and more than willing to give me his undivided attention. When I mentioned that I had been taking antibiotics, he seemed surprised. I soon discovered that he had never treated patients with antibiotics. He was, however, quick to declare that he held Dr. Trentham in high regard. I tried to hide my chagrin. How could this happen? It had taken me over a month to get an appointment. Now I was back to square one —no *Road Back* rheumatologist, no hand surgeon, and my joints were getting worse.

On the *Road Back* homepage I soon discovered that the shuffle, delay, rebuke, and confusion I was experiencing were common for rheumatoid patients. Much of the problem lies in deteriorating health economics and restrictive insurance coverage that prevent doctors from giving complicated chronic illnesses the time and attention they deserve, including time spent communicating with a patient's other doctors. In the midst of the muddle, memory fails, mistakes are made, and those with serious problems are commonly neglected and grow disheartened. Only the extremely wealthy patients who can opt out of the insurance system and afford pricey individual care, have much chance of avoiding the shuffle and confusion.

The problems are especially exasperating if you are seeking anything other than off-the-shelf medicine. Awareness of alternative therapies is rare among conventionally trained rheumatologists. Until the late 1990s, only a small minority were familiar with the antibiotic protocol despite the fact that it had been practiced for fifty years and was supported by considerable research.

On the *Road Back* and related web sites, stories abound of suffering rheumatoid patients taking years to gain an accurate diagnosis. By the time they discover that mycoplasma might play some role in their disease, they may have undergone several joint operations and suffered the side effects of many toxic drugs. The problem is exacerbated by the fact that rheumatoid problems cross so many disciplines. For my rheumatoid disease, psoriatic arthritis, I was potentially looking at nineteen medical specialties for the treatment of at least fifteen different problems.

Rheumatic Problems and Related Health Specialties

1. **Joint Inflammation:** *Rheumatology; Orthopedics*
2. **Metabolism, Energy and Adrenals:** *Internal Medicine; Endocrinology; Acupuncture; Naturopathy*
3. **Fibromyalgia:** *Internal Medicine; Endocrinology; Naturopathy; Acupuncture*
4. **Hands:** *Hand Orthopedics; Hand Occupational Therapy*
5. **Feet:** *Foot and Ankle Orthopedics; Foot Occupational Therapy*
6. **Urinary and Prostate:** *Urology*
7. **Digestion and Nutrition:** *Gastroenterology; Internal Medicine; Naturopathy*
8. **Skin and Nails:** *Dermatology; Rheumatology; Internal Medicine*
9. **Depression:** *Psychiatry; Psychology; Acupuncture*
10. **Back, Knees, Hips and Other Joints:** *Orthopedics; Physical Therapy; Rheumatology, Acupuncture, Osteopathy, Chiropractic*
11. **Sleep Disorders**: *Endocrinology; Internal Medicine; Naturopathy*
12. **Vision:** *Ophthalmology*
13. **Allergies**: *Allergies; Internal Medicine; Naturopathy*
14. **Breathing:** *Internal Medicine, Cardiology, Emergency Medicine*
15. **Heart and Arteries:** *Cardiology; Emergency Medicine*

The complexity of the various rheumatoid disorders is such that the eruption of a problem in one area often triggers complications in another. For example, thyroid and adrenals can be imbalanced by inflammation, sleep deficit, poor nutrition, and persistently acute stress. However, backward and forward causality confounds the system of relationships. When adrenals are overloaded, natural cortisol is eventually depleted which may spike inflammation and provoke fatigue and sleep-cycle disruption. These, in turn, can lead to poor digestion, sluggish liver, and reduced clearance of toxins by the lymph system, all of which can amplify other disorders. As a result, rheumatoid patients often feel that they are caught up in an inexorable whirlpool.

Medications often exacerbate and speed up the spiral. In taking antibiotics to deal with opportunistic microbes, a person can easily kill off beneficial gut flora. This can lead to leaky gut and further microbe invasion of the bloodstream. Steroids and NSAIDs (non-steroidal anti-inflammatory drugs) may dampen inflammation but worsen leaky gut and this may lead to even more inflammation. Taking prednisone at more than small doses can lead to swelling and edema, high blood pressure, muscle weakness, increased susceptibility to infection, mood swings, and depression.

In most cases, each symptom in the syndrome is treated separately with little consideration of complications across specialties. This is particularly true if the patient is being seen for an acute problem or for a surgery. My own experience was that most specialists, whether seeing me for joint problems, adrenals, thyroid, mouth sores, inflamed knees, or dizziness, weren't particularly interested in the fact that psoriatic arthritis was the central problem and itself might be caused by infection. Whenever I brought this up, I got no more than a dismissive shrug. It seemed that I was volunteering something irrelevant. I never had the feeling that it had any bearing on what was prescribed, though I knew that my system was highly sensitive to any change of regimen.

In mid 2002, I realized an important coup when I discovered Carol Nicholson, a talented occupational therapist who began helping me control my hand inflammation. First, she attacked the swelling by devising a rigorous protocol that consisted of hot and cold soaking. We then experimented with pressure compresses that helped even more. When the swelling subsided, we began working on exercises to increase range of motion. The exercises made use of several customized dynamic splints that took careful account of my problem tendons and ligaments. What I appreciated most about Carol was her curiosity and inventiveness. She seemed to enjoy the challenge of every problem and in my mind, epitomized the explorer mentality I had written about in *The Mindful Traveler*.

Nearing the end of summer 2002, the hand therapy had clearly helped and possibly the use of brand minocycline as well. It was now less painful to work at my computer and execute simple daily chores like doing dishes and opening cans and bottles. This coincided with a reduction in my morning dizziness. The fog seemed to have lifted on the Golden Gate or at least the captain wasn't teetering around drunk in the pilothouse. For this, I was most grateful.

As my condition improved, I began paying more attention to the outside world. On a frequent basis, I replied to postings on the *Road Back* bulletin board, trying to help others by passing on information I had come across in my own research. It felt good to help, but I often felt that people simply wanted me to tell them what to do.

In Dire Straits

I didn't want to do that. I was under no illusion that I was an expert, just someone who had done the work to understand the science and the uncertainties, and to ask the right questions. I also believed that getting well usually required some amount of self-empowerment. Otherwise, as soon as a remedy lost effectiveness, you would be back in the same position of not knowing where to turn and what to do. Sadly, the most desperate people bounced from one person's advice to next, never really paying attention to what might explain their response and what their best options were.

This reminded me of how rudderless and grasping my own mom had been when stricken with lymphoma. She didn't really believe that she could make the right decisions or even ask the right questions, so she placed all her faith in doctors whom she largely selected based on demeanor, rather than substance. I'm sure she would have been more thoughtful and discerning if she had been less terrified and drugged. However, she passed that point early on by taking high doses of steroids and mind-altering drugs.

Now people seemed to be grasping for my help in the same way—with no critical discrimination or healthy objectivity. Even if you offered caveats, they usually went unheeded.

In early fall of 2002, my concern about swollen joints was giving way to apprehension about the inflamed world and the rising rhetoric of war. Claims of impending peril from Iraq's alleged arsenal of chemical, biological, and nuclear weapons were stirring support for a pre-emptive invasion, even among people I considered thoughtful and informed.

Nearly every day, someone from the Bush Administration or connections with Drudge, Fox News, or *The Weekly Standard*, was beating the war drum, suggesting links between Saddam and terrorists, or making unsupported assertions that weapons inspections had failed miserably and represented US government entitlement to enforce UN resolutions.

On October 7, George Bush stated, "The evidence indicates that Iraq is reconstituting its nuclear weapons program...Iraq has attempted to purchase high-strength aluminum tubes and other equipment needed for gas centrifuges, which are used to enrich uranium for nuclear weapons." On the same day he added, "We have also discovered through intelligence that Iraq has a growing fleet of manned and unmanned aerial vehicles (UAVs) that could be used to disperse chemical or biological weapons across broad areas. We are concerned that Iraq is exploring ways of using these UAVs for missions targeting the United States."

Buddha, who heard the same remark, blurted out, "They're targeting the US with model airplanes?"

"Apparently they're planning to fly them in from Iraq," I answered.

It was clear that the Bush Administration was agitating the wild elephant and pointing him in the direction of Iraq. With my newfound energy and joint mobility, I decided to do even more to stop the rush to war. I was soon scouring the daily papers, keeping track of the most outrageous claims and composing letters and essays and articles to counter and refute the nonsense. My distribution net included web pages, my circle of old college friends, the local papers, various newsletters, and a progressive talk show host, who seemed to appreciate my contributions and suggestions.

What mystified me most was that the mainstream media seemed so ready to accept and pass on what they were told by government sources and the Iraqi National Congress, the group headed by Ahmed Chalabi. Judith Miller, the international reporter for the *New York Times*, repeatedly conveyed threat information without offering provisos and qualifications. It was as if the *Times* had become a propaganda arm of the government and was most happy to pass on the steroidal soma to the general population. I was sure that if Miller ever decided to switch careers she would have no trouble landing a job in the PR division of one of the major pharmaceutical companies, perhaps the steroids division.

Buddha was having particular difficulty getting over his confusion about the UAV threat. "I used to have a model Flying Tiger in my youth," he declared in his undulating Indian accent. "Do you suppose this is the kind of UAV they are talking about? Maybe Saddam plans to launch them from Mexico, or Canada, or from the fleet of Iraqi nuclear submarines. But then again, maybe he will refuel them with tanker models. These Iraqis appear to be crackerjack scientists. Let's only hope that they don't begin experimenting with Tesla death rays."

On November 17, 2003, Calvin Trillin, the *New Yorker* satirist, imagined a press conference interrogation of George Bush by a Zen reporter. We were quite sure that this had already taken place in Kathmandu almost a year earlier.

This penchant for asking the wrong questions probably explained why so few Buddhist and Zen reporters were called on at White House press conferences. They couldn't be trusted anymore than I could be trusted by the community of Seattle hand surgeons.

Excerpt from George Bush's Press Conference in Kathmandu

Zen Monk: "Sir, if the ability of the Star Wars ABMs to hit a nuclear missile is imaginary and nuclear missiles in Iraq are imaginary, does that mean a Star Wars ABM could hit an Iraqi nuclear missile?"

Source: *The New Yorker*, November 17, 2003

In December 2002, I listened to an audio by a former marine who dissected every important administration claim regarding weapons of mass destruction. Although I was struck by his meticulous detail and point-by-point rigor, what impressed me most was how he linked use of propaganda to violation of the Constitution. He noted that when soldiers, marines, airmen, and sailors signed up for the service, they took an oath to defend the Constitution. The President and Vice President were bound by this as well. In his mind, an elected leader who took the nation to war on the basis of a lie was allowing ends to justify means and this was antithetical to the Constitution and the rule of law. Few crimes against the people were so serious and offensive as this.

I thought about this for several days. It seemed to capsulate my objection to the war. There could be any number of justifications for going to war—to stop war crimes, to defend against an attack, and maybe even to prevent a planned attack, but on Constitutional and moral grounds, you couldn't go to war on the basis of a grossly exaggerated threat or a lie, and one or the other was clearly at play here. After all, the UN weapons inspectors, including Hans Blix, were stating that almost all the WMD were accounted for and with only a few months more work, verification would be complete. Despite this, the Administration ordered the inspectors out. Something was seriously wrong here.

In the rush to war, few people seemed willing to consider the hard and documented evidence of threat, the consequences, or side effects of the steroidal anti-inflammatory fix. There were a few, however, including General Shinseki who was quickly marginalized for arguing that the war would require several hundred thousand men. Other retired CIA officials, including Ray McGovern and Greg Thielmann, disputed the claims that Iraq possessed WMD that could threaten the US and charged that Administration was distorting intelligence and using it for political purposes. Together they personified the enlightened warriors I had written about in *The Mindful Traveler*. These were people who believed that the reasons for war mattered, the Geneva Convention mattered, and that ends alone didn't justify the means.

The code was perhaps best reflected by the story of Arjuna in the Bhagavad Gita, who refused simply to take up arms because it was expected of him.

I was still thinking about this when I learned that the Jain monk and peace activist, Satish Kumar, was scheduled to give a talk at the Chinook Institute, located on Whidbey Island northwest of Seattle. Satish gained notice in 1963 by protesting nuclear proliferation with an eight thousand-mile peace walk. The walk began in India and passed through Moscow, Paris, London, and Washington D.C. Like King and Gandhi, Satish was a skilled practitioner of non-violent disobedience. In his peace-walk he stirred world opinion and the anxiety of world leaders simply by arriving at the corridors of power with teabags that symbolized world peace.

In the Soviet Union, the President of the Supreme Soviet recognized the danger of adverse publicity and went out of his way to expedite Satish's passage to the West. Air transportation was arranged, but on March 13, 1963, Satish simply walked out of his Moscow room and pointed in the direction of Poland. After arriving in Paris several months later, he indiscreetly spoke out against French nuclear tests in the South Pacific, which landed him in a filthy jail. The resulting public outcry caused the French authorities to reconsider their inhospitality and speed him on his way to Britain.

Soon arriving in London, he asked for an audience with Prime Minister Harold Wilson. A meeting with such a lowly Indian was not possible, but the eminent Lord Atlee cordially accepted the teabag on the Prime Minister's behalf, in the process explaining that disarmament was being blocked by the Russians, who were the real threat to world peace. Satish's counter-arguments were cordially accepted and he was politely offered Godspeed on the last leg of his journey to America.

Crossing to the United States aboard the *Queen Mary*, Satish arrived in New York and then walked to Washington, D.C. His original hope was to deliver a teabag to John

Kennedy but Lyndon Johnson was now in office. In Johnson's place, the teabag was accepted by an arms negotiator, who not surprisingly explained that disarmament was impeded by others possessing evil intent.

I first met Satish at a transpersonal psychology conference in Killarney, Ireland in 1994. In subsequent years, I visited him at Schumacher College where he was programme director, and then later acted as his chauffeur on a tour for his book, *Path Without Destination*. In 2000, he provided a thoughtful cover testimonial for *The Mindful Traveler*. Beyond simply renewing our connection, I looked forward to his thoughts about the rush to war and perhaps some insights on the way of the enlightened warrior in a time of mass frenzy. It was a trying and difficult time for spirit and I could certainly use a dose of his gentle wisdom.

Chapter 8

Walking with Satish

To reach the Chinook Center on Whidbey Island required a one-hour drive and a half-hour ferry connection across Puget Sound. The journey itself was a welcomed change of routine, particularly the ferry ride, which renewed my appreciation of the natural wonder and beauty of Puget Sound, which I hadn't paid much attention to since the onset of my illness. The center was located on a spacious parcel of timberland on the south part of the island and largely undeveloped except for walking paths through the woods, several peripheral log cabins, and a central conference hall constructed from stone and prime timber. As I made my way along the path from the parking lot to the main building, I could hear the sweep of great evergreen boughs in the misty breeze. I was quite sure Satish must have noticed this as well on his own arrival. He was a most observant walker and a deep listener when it came to the natural environment.

When I had been his Seattle chauffeur in 1998, I had taken him on a walk to the city's oldest evergreen tree. Along the way he stopped to take in the scent of ferns and

In Dire Straits

wildflowers and to commune with songbirds.

Deep Listening

But he learned more from the river than Vasudeva could teach him. He learned from it continually. Above all, he learned from it how to listen with a still heart, with a waiting open soul, without passion, without desire, without judgement, without opinions.

Source: *Siddhartha*, Hermann Hesse

Even before I reached the front porch of the main building, I could tell from the buzz that a formidable crowd had gathered, which was all the more impressive given the distance from Seattle and other major cities. More impressive still, this was a Sunday evening in the middle of winter. I was sure that the turnout had something to do with the fact that people were hoping for his insights during this time of worldwide crisis.

I found a seat at the back of the packed conference room and listened as the director introduced him. Satish appeared smiling and immediately the faces brightened around me. He always worked this kind of effect on the people he spoke to. Crows feet framed his penetrating brown eyes. A small and wiry man of perhaps five feet seven, 140 pounds, his manner belied his age. He was in his sixties but carried himself like a person of forty. He exuded fitness, but of course he was an inveterate walker. No telling how many miles he had logged in just the last week. I was quite sure that it exceeded my own yearly total, even before the arthritis.

"It is always good to come to the Northwest and this

96

wonderful retreat here in the woods on Whidbey Island. It is quite renewing don't you think? A very good place to take a long walk."

"I would like to tell you about walking," he declared ebulliently. "It can be quite helpful in times like these. I learned to walk from my mother and discovered many lessons along the way. When I was born, a Brahmin in my Indian village told my mother that I would be a child of unfulfilled wishes and that I would never reach my destination." He chuckled and shrugged and the audience seemed to register on the allusion to his book, *Path Without Destination.*

He began talking about the sensory delights of walking —there was much more to walking than one usually imagined. In every footfall there were different sensations that depended on the terrain—the rebound off unyielding surfaces, the slide across gravel, cushioned softness of fir needles, such as those along the forested path from the parking lot. "New discoveries are everywhere to be found along the way, but in order to perceive them, one must still an anxious mind and dispense with many expectations."

As he continued to describe the sensations of walking, I realized that my own focus had changed dramatically in two years. My own basin and range had contracted dramatically and, as a result, I was now visited by different sights and sounds from morning to sunset. Just a few years ago, as a professional ecologist, I frequently waded through streams and grassy wetlands perked to the rustling of voles or the shriek of red-tailed hawks.

Because I now spent so much time in bed or in the tub,

my ears had grown accustomed to domestic, urban sounds. I knew the cresting fugue of the freeways that began at 5 a.m. In mid-evening, before sunset, came the double-pitched cries of the varied thrush in my backyard, and then in the early a.m., the madding rat-tat-tat of a sapsucker in a high spruce tree next to my bedroom window. That single bird ruined the warm embrace of tearless dreams and drove me to the edge of violent retribution. But Buddha came to his rescue with a message of *ahimsa*, and I turned the torment into a sleepy-time mantra. Satish would have been proud of me for that.

Nonviolence (Ahimsa)

Ahimsa, or nonviolence, is a universal first principle of non-offensive living. Hindus, Buddhists, Jains, Jews, Muslims, Christians, and followers of all other religions, one way or another, have to a greater or lesser extent proclaimed this to be fundamental. Nonviolence should underlie all relationships among humans and between humans and the nonhuman world. Nonviolence is a part of the the Perennial Philosophy. But Gandhi made it more relevant to our time by using it as a weapon of resistance to social injustice, to British colonialism, to economic exploitation of the weak by the strong, to caste discrimination in India.

Source: *Path Without Destination*, Satish Kumar

I had also become an expert on the percussion of rushing water—not the waterfalls of the Snoqualmie or Skagit rivers as I had in earlier years, but the torrent of tap water filling my tub, and then cycling around my feeble joints like an orphaned Charybdis.

There was even playfulness in my domestic hydrology that fulminated from an under-employed mind. I posed the seminal question that Archimedes somehow missed: when the water grows tepid, can you warm it more quickly by cranking the tap or by first allowing some of the lukewarm water to drain? Buddha as Thinker took this way too seriously, blurting out a differential equation, which provoked hooting and catcalls from Buffy, the other dolls, and my two main teddy bears, Schoomer and Big Sydney.

I wondered whether Satish had surrendered to such idle whimsy in those endless hill-climbs through The Khyber Pass and Uzbekistan and the deadening monotony of the Polish flatland.

He had shifted to the matter of balance: it was important to walk with economy, with limited yet relaxed motion in both upper and lower body: you might even say all the chakras were engaged in a balanced walk. "And breath is most important—it is very easy to fall into shallow breathing which robs the mind and body. Be full and joyful in your breathing—take a generous drink from the cup." He took a deep breath and the audience heaved a collective sigh like a great whale intoxicated with its own ambergris.

"There are always questions about gait and stride and proper rhythm. Gandhi spoke of walking with two legs: on one leg you create the alternative society; on the other you confront obstruction to change. Vinoba, who walked with Gandhi to create land reform in India, felt that opposition is only counter-productive because it stirs defensiveness. He believed in patience and the gentle moral appeal. Of course, in India, time is not viewed as a problem. There are many turnings of the wheel. Still, it is a difficult question if you remain concerned about injustice and suffering."

Satish left it to you to read between the lines, to find your own equilibrium between hot and cold, between draining the tub and turning the tap, or simply getting out of the tub and walking away. It was the art of the Zen master, the Hindu Brahmin, and the Tibetan rinpoche to provoke with questions and musings rather than deliver a hammer blow of insight.

I couldn't help but think of the Bhagavad Gita, one of the great Hindu holy books, whose dialogue revolves around the struggles of conscience for Arjuna, the thoughtful warrior, who is verged on taking up arms in a bloody family struggle. His master and charioteer, Krishna, asks the difficult questions and provokes Arjuna to explore higher self or *Atman*.

"I try to walk with both legs, like Gandhi, and not get too bouncy," Satish declared.

"Such perfect simplicity, calming as well as centering. You become an example to others."

It was no wonder that Satish caused such a ruckus by presenting his teabags to the world powers. He was right: delivering a teabag in the right manner could change the world.

"Fearlessness is the greatest challenge," he offered. "Fear is the cause of aggression and violence. Because of fear, we want to control, dominate, and rule others. Fear erodes personal as well as social harmony. The cure for the problems created by fear is unconditional trust in the workings of the universe. As we trust that the sun will rise, water will quench thirst, fire will cook food, boats will sail the seas, so we have to trust that each life, including our own, will fulfill its destiny.

Walking is very good for trust."

He noted that before embarking on his long-distance walk, he and his mate were counseled by Vinoba to take no money. This would open them up to the generosity and good will of others, and so it did. Everyone wanted to help by offering meals and clothing, shelter and water. Even the militant Muslims and tribal warriors in Afghanistan welcomed them as honored guests. Satish paused for people to absorb the significance of this. I wished that someone could send that pause to George Bush or Donald Rumsfeld.

He ended with a message about truth or the Indian concept of *satya*. It was closely related to trust. Even when you were on a truthful path, uncertainty was unavoidable. There would always be lapses in confidence because reality was chimerical. But these could be addressed. Certainty and direction could be restored by remaining open and committed "to face things as they are. Quite often, very interesting discoveries will come around the bend."

He bowed humbly and was immediately deluged with applause and surrounded by well-wishers. I hoped to talk to him, but I could see that this would be difficult. A score of people seemed to be waiting. A bit disappointed, I headed for the cafeteria to see if I could purchase a supplemental ticket for dinner. I waited in line for several minutes and then decided I wasn't that hungry. As I turned away contemplating my return home, I noticed Satish at the front door. He was alone and staring into the surrounding forest. I hesitated and approached him, not quite sure if he would recognize me. Though we had talked by phone, I hadn't seen him for two years.

"How good to see you, Jim," he declared with a warm handshake. "Are you still restoring the life of water?"

It took me a moment to realize what he was talking about. When I last visited him in England, he had invited me to lunch and asked me about my work. I told him that I had been working with a group of scientists at the Pacific Watershed Institute on an integrated and unusual approach to protecting watersheds. When I later purchased a copy of his book, he inscribed it with the words, "With love and gratitude for the work you do to restore the life of water."

"The institute dissolved, but I never get too far away from water these days," I answered.

"Perhaps you would like to take a short walk with me?"

"Yes, of course, if you have the time. You might miss dinner."

He shrugged and opened the door ahead of me.

We walked into the blustery wind and I hoped that I could keep up with him. "Yes, I am very glad to see you," I blurted out.

"And your book is continuing to do well?"

"I haven't checked of late but I'm afraid that the decline in travel will have an effect. On the bright side, I much enjoy the talks and meetings with international travelers."

"Yes, that is always a delight. And you are continuing to write?"

I nodded.

"You must come to Schumacher," he declared.

"I would love that," I thought of telling him about my

health problems but knew it would divert the discussion. For the moment we simply walked, tracing a shallow outward arc toward the distant property line. Despite my slight limp, we fell into a relaxed concinnity of pace that reminded me of our first walk together to Seattle's patriarch evergreen. In the deep woods we remained silent, taking in the groan of tree limbs, the dripping of moisture into forest puddles, and the occasional, high-pitched fribitt of a Pacific tree frog. Satish's face was printed with serene delight.

Soon we emerged in the open and he wanted to know more about my work. I was a little embarrassed, answering in abstracts that hardly disguised my recent indolence. He seemed to want more so I told him that I had been reading and writing about grief and attachment, and these seemed to relate to my own health and the state of the world, and suddenly he was nodding intently, as if I had said something significant, or more likely, that a rare pygmy owl had just streaked above my head and landed on a nearby perch. No, there didn't seem to be any owl, but I decided not to ruin the illusion and simply added: "I haven't quite worked it out." That seemed to satisfy him so we simply walked.

When we returned to the main building, he declared that it had been a delightful respite—exactly what he hoped for and with just the right person. I flushed with appreciation and gave him a parting hug. As I backed away down the trail, he declared that I should contact him in a month or two before coming to the college. "We have a good library," he cried out from afar.

I wasn't exactly sure about this offer. Was it to be taken

seriously? There couldn't be a better place to work on a book than Schumacher College, that is, if you had a book to write. Maybe he was just inviting me to drop in for a day or two as I had when I was last in England. That probably made more sense. Either way, it was very flattering that he would show such interest in me.

On the ferry home, I replayed portions of the lecture and then the dialogue in the woods, and it almost seemed like an extension of the Gita. It was hard to miss the message in his talk that any person, even a lowly Indian, was capable of making a difference, if somehow they could surmount their fears and begin their peace walk. He insisted that his only real gift was a good set of legs and that was all he really needed to deliver his teabags.

Of course, I knew that was only part of it. It was hard to think of another traveler surrounded by as many Buddhas as Satish. First and foremost, he was the rarest of communicators. Even at the Killarney Conference in 1994, populated by the likes of Ram Dass, Jack Kornfield, Peter Russell, Christina and Stanislav Grof, he stole the show with his simple talk on walking, much like the one he had just delivered. He was obviously both a healer and warrior, but maybe even more than this, personified Buddha as Mystic. In fact, I could imagine few others who so well demonstrated these many qualities.

Up until now it hadn't quite dawned on me that trust and fearlessness provided an underlying substrate for both the credo and the curiosities of the mystic. They combined to create the kind of openness that invited inspiration, amazing synchronicities, and siddhi-like powers. It was no wonder that the British Empire crumbled under the assault of powers like this. A Jain waif bearing a teabag could be far more dangerous than any brigade of infantry or the deafening barrage of the largest siege guns. It was the shock and awe of perfect silence.

Credo and Curiosities of Buddha as Mystic

Credo and Mindset
1. I can transcend ego.
2. I can realize higher self.
3. I can quell my negative internal chatter through reflection, meditation and mindfulness.
4. I am more than my body, more than what I do, more than what I create, and more than what I think.
5. I can be of service to others.
6. I can find joy in being, discovery, expression and service.
7. Overboard with the baggage.
8. I am grateful.

Questions and Curiosities
1. What are my blind spots?
2. What are my voices of limitation and how do I transcend them?
3. In what ways can I be of service to others?
4. In what ways am I connected to others?
5. Where is the path with heart?

Source: *The Mindful Traveler* (Open Court, 2000)

Perhaps I would do something similar. Maybe a walk to Washington, D.C., to stop the war. I didn't have teabags, but I would come up with something appropriate. I would trust the universe to provide the perfect gift for George Bush.

At once, five different Buddha shouted out, "Are you nuts? When was the last time you checked your feet and knees? How long do you think they would hold up? The end of the first block? Maybe we should try to make it to the local café in the morning before taking on a 3,500 mile march." I had to admit this made some sense. In fact, my feet were killing me after the long walk in the woods. I was going to need several days to recover.

I fell into deeper thought about what I might contribute to the anti-war effort. I would leave the marching and peace walks to others. Perhaps I could make some public presentations. Yes, that was a possibility, except for the fact that my travel talks seldom drew a large audience. Then, too, it wouldn't exactly be easy to make the leap from the vicissitudes of travel to the phony links between Saddam and 9/11. No, I would leave the public rejoinders to Ray McGovern, Greg Thielmann, and the other enlightened warriors.

I did have one skill that I could tap, and Satish had reminded me of that—I could write and could integrate the important points of others. Maybe I could put that to good use. Perhaps I could monitor and expose the Orwellian propaganda and bring it to the attention of others who might already have misgivings about the war. It wasn't necessary to publish articles in *The Nation, The New Yorker,* or *The New York Times*. I needed only to reach my own circle of friends and acquaintances. They, in turn, could pass on the articles to their own contacts. That was the beauty of the web.

Maybe I could also invoke Buddha as Harlequin to take up the cause. Satire was one of the best ways to reach people —that and good performance art. I had a few rebellious artist friends who could be counted on for some outrageous Dada. In the meantime, I needed to get to work, scour the best papers, and collect information to show the legal and moral indefensibility of the invasion.

For several months I wrote essays, satire, and open public letters on everything from Iraq's weapons capabilities to the workings of the Office of Special Plans in the Pentagon. I wrote about the Neocon philosophy and its dangers to democracy and I collated and distributed the opinions of Ray McGovern and other enlightened warriors about the corruption and distortion of war intelligence by the White House.

More time-consuming efforts carried me into the realm of physics and medicine. I stated the case against depleted uranium munitions, drawing on studies and anecdotal information from the First Gulf War. Then I bridged to the data available on autoimmune diseases experienced by veterans on their return home. There was an alarming case to be made that the dangers of the upcoming Gulf war would be far greater than the first.

My main outlet was the homepage of my Harvard College class, but on a regular basis I also submitted letters to the editor of local papers, sent off e-mail to friends, and submitted essays to magazines and newsletters. It wasn't brilliant and original material, but my intent wasn't to win rave critical reviews, only to circulate a story that wasn't widely being told and to jog people to consider more deeply what they were hearing and reading. I wouldn't have taken this on if the major networks and newspapers had been doing their jobs.

As I put together the information, I kept returning to what Morris Berman had said in the *Twilight of American*

In Dire Straits

Culture about the dumbing-down of American society. I really was beginning to wonder whether most Americans had lost the ability to discriminate, and if so, how it had come about. Why were they so susceptible to propaganda? Was it the education system or the dimming effects of fear, the same very response I had seen on the *Road Back* homepage from people in distress who flailed about looking for an authoritative voice that would rescue them from their pain and suffering?

Chapter 9

Chinatown

Until January of 2003, I had hoped to avoid joint replacement for the worst finger on my right hand with a delicate joint replacement, but I lost hope of that at about the time that George Bush appeared before Congress in his 2003 State of the Union Message and recited the dangers of a WMD-fortified Iraq with connections to terrorist groups.

In early 2002, a qualified surgeon in north Seattle rejected me for no particular reason. After a bit of sleuthing, I discovered that he had received some sort of warning about me from an unnamed hand surgeon at another clinic. I appealed to him to reconsider, but he was unmoved. I then rang up Carol Nicholson again and she gave me another name. Unfortunately, this doctor was a younger associate of the head doctor at the Formalin clinic, who wouldn't allow anyone else in his clinic to see me.

I was more concerned than angry. I was rapidly running out of Seattle hand surgeons. All of them seemed to be networked and sharing the same intelligence that apparently rated me as a threat to the established order.

In Dire Straits

In mid 2002, about the time that CBS broke the story on George Bush receiving a daily brief on the danger of hijackers flying planes into buildings, it occurred to me that I possessed all the material for a really impressive conspiracy theory. Dick Cheney and George Tenet had clearly joined forces with the entire Seattle Society of Hand Surgeons who were trying to link me to a meeting with Mohammed Atta in Prague, cover up intelligence on the 9/11 attacks as well as the true reasons for the collapse of Trade Tower Building C.

Far-fetched imagination kept my spirits up. In February 2003, I was finally able to exhale when I found a board-certified hand surgeon willing to operate on me. Just prior to the pre-op appointment, I met with Madeleine. She suggested that I again draft a series of detailed questions, among other things making sure that I knew what kind of anesthetic would be used. She, too, had graduated summa cum laude from the Ralph Golan School of Patient Assertiveness.

She was quick to relate another story from her doctor friend Maury. Maury was skeptic about almost all general anesthesia and as a patient hardly ever consented to it. Apparently during pre-op for his recent colonoscopy he informed the surgical nurse that he wanted neither a general nor a local—"none whatsoever." The nurse answered that she didn't feel "comfortable with that" and was quite sure that the doctor wouldn't sanction it. Maury's reply was succinct and emphatic: "You don't feel comfortable with it? You *get* comfortable with it or find someone that can." It made me think of the famous Seinfeld episode in which George learns that Jerry has spent the night with Elaine and Jerry refuses to offer details.

"No details? …You listen to me and you listen to me good—I want details and I want them now."

Madeleine didn't seem to understand my situation. Yes, I was concerned that the anesthetic might affect my immune system, but this might be the only surgeon left in Seattle who would operate on me. "I don't think giving orders is in the cards for me. Remember whom you're talking to: I'm not a retired gynecologist from New York. I'm on the medical watch list, along with Uday and Qusay."

My initial meeting with Dr. West came on the eve of the Baghdad Shock and Awe. Dr. West was congenial and composed. He seemed impressed by my reticence and willingness to defer to his expertise. Seeing as I had few questions of my own, he figured I might want to know that the joint fusion would take about an hour. My finger and adjacent ones would then be immobilized in a temporary splint. A few weeks later the splint would be replaced by a cast, which would remain in place for a month.

"I'm sure you'll do a good job, doc," I answered biting my tongue and silently chanting, "Ohm, Mani Padme Hum."

The April 3 operation seemed to go well. A few hours after I arrived home, I learned that the Third Infantry Division had poured through the Karbala Gap in an unimpeded run to Baghdad. The evening news described this in terms reminiscent of the breakout from Normandy. The only mention of anyone dying related to the report of an Iraqi division being eviscerated to the northeast. When the footage came up of the destruction and dead bodies, I reached for my bottle of

Percocet.

In those first few days of medicated, narcotic ecstasy, it came to me that so much of my life had been a joyless struggle against authority—environmental, political, and even professional. More often I needed to let go, the way I had at the hospital, the way I had at that pre-op meeting with Dr. West. Life could be so much easier if I could muster some degree of trust.

A week passed and Dr. West replaced my small cast with a bulkier one. Then fatigue set in. It wasn't an ordinary fatigue, but the kind that brought giants to their knees. It rivaled the severity of the near-coma I experienced after my mom died. I was only functional for five or six hours a day, usually in the late evening and early morning.

Madeleine said she had heard similar stories of people having trouble bouncing back after operations, especially when they had been given general anesthetics.

I wasn't quite ready to admit it, but maybe I hadn't asked enough questions.

There was another worry that was even more troubling —that the operation or the anesthetic had worsened my arthritis. Dr. Brown talked about fatigue as an indication that mycoplasma might be migrating, perhaps escaping from joints where it had been encased by inflammation. If it were spreading, it might be finding a new home in my knees, neck, and lower back, all of which were now sensitive or aching.

My spirits received another blow when the cast came off and I discovered that my finger had been set at thirty degrees. This was a much steeper angle than Dr. West and I had talked about. It would clearly make it difficult for me to play sports, especially basketball. I guess I was still holding out hope that eventually I would recover to the point that basketball was still possible.

I mentioned my disappointment to Madeleine. but she didn't seem to grasp my dismay. For me, basketball had always been more than exercise. It was a form of exuberant expression and an outlet for stress. It had gotten me through any number of life crises, including failed relationships, rejected manuscripts, and even my mom's death. I guess you had to be a basketball junkie to understand something like this.

I did know one person who would understand—my long-time friend, Mel, with whom I had played basketball since my twenties. At the same time, I knew I had to be a little careful in fishing for his sympathy. He had always been the sort of person who believed that if someone knocked your nose off with their elbow, you simply taped it back on and replied in kind.

"I just don't see how I'll ever be able to shoot again. I can't even extend my fingers."

He shrugged and quickly replied, "Get used to playing defense. You never could shoot anyway." The laugh made me feel a little better.

Madeleine came up with another compensation I hadn't thought of: my crooked thirty-degree digit made it look as though I were giving someone the finger. That might come in handy as an appropriate gesture in my harangues about the Neocons and the unconstitutional Iraq war.

Despite the many attempts to slough off my difficulties

as temporary, my symptoms only seemed to be worsening. My left shoulder was killing me, my hip was aching, my knees were throbbing, and I could no longer bend another finger that had been immobilized for six weeks in my cast to protect the fused joint. When I showed Carol Nicholson my hand and explained what had happened, she erupted—she couldn't imagine that a hand surgeon would immobilize my other fingers for six weeks when he knew that my arthritis was so aggressive: the results were obvious and predictable. She fitted me with a new dynamic splint to see if we could loosen up the frozen joint and I began a search for something that would slow down my overall disease process.

Doctor Brown had suggested that histamines sometimes surround infected cells and prevent antibiotics from clearing an intercellular infection. He had occasionally used Benadryl to penetrate the screen. I decided to add it as well as quercitin (a natural antihistamine) to my weekly antibiotic regimen. I noticed no immediate improvement, but I didn't expect a quick response.

Searching for some new possibility of my downturn, I scheduled a meeting with my new primary care doctor to see if she could help. It was the first time I had seen her since before my operation. As soon as she set eyes on me she was concerned: apparently my skin tone was wan and my eyes were glassy and listless. She was particularly concerned when I told her of my extreme fatigue. She figured I might be suffering from hypothyroidism, and that this was symptomatic of the progression of the disease. In her opinion I needed to see a rheumatologist as soon as possible.

I said I would consider seeing one, but as far as I knew, there was no one in the area who believed in the therapy I was following, and I still wasn't ready to take immune-system suppressants. She didn't argue, but I could tell that she thought I was making a mistake in being so stubborn and really ought to quit playing doctor.

In the aftermath, I felt increasingly isolated and alone on the healing path that I had chosen. On a daily basis, I asked myself whether I *was* being stubborn and irrational, but every time I conducted the interrogation, I only convinced myself that I was doing the right thing in refusing a path that would lead to immune suppression. Eventually there might be a point in considering the new designer drugs, such as Enbrel and Remicade, but the case for them still wasn't as convincing as that for antibiotics, especially given the fact that I had tested positive for mycoplasma. Perhaps more important, I knew that my current treatment was not putting me at risk for toxic side-effects.

It was a time, I believed, to dig in and show some resolve, to show even more discipline in my diet and commitment to a soft path in healing myself. I became even more resolute in embracing the warrior credo of *The Mindful Traveler*.

In my moments of eroding self-confidence, I took courage from the unwavering resoluteness of Ray McGovern, Greg Thielmann, and other enlightened warriors opposing the war. The statue of Saddam had been torn down and the pseudo-patriots were regaling in the fall of Baghdad, but the enlightened warriors were relentless in reminding the press of the expressed reasons for war and the fact that the Bush Administration was changing its rationale. First it was the WMD, then the sadism of Saddam, then creating a democracy in Iraq.

Because of my sleep problems, I was becoming a night owl, and nearly every night listened to a provocative talk show, hosted by the outspoken Seattle Progressive, Mike Webb. He frequently interviewed Ray McGovern, Greg Thielmann, Joseph Wilson, Al Franken, Arianna Huffington, and other critics of the war, raising questions you didn't normally hear on talk radio: Where are the weapons? How and why is the story changing? What is the background of these chickenhawks who are so quick to promote military intervention and pre-emptive strikes?

With my limited energies I researched topics related to the war and passed on the results to Mike. These included the harmful effects of depleted uranium and the data on Gulf War Syndrome. I also alerted him to the outing of Joseph Wilson's wife by someone within the White House (first aired in Seattle on his program), and submitted a list of questions for an interview of Greg Thielmann, the heroic ex-State Department employee who reported on the cherrypicking of intelligence by the Pentagon Office of Special Plans.

It felt good to be making a small contribution to the anti-war effort, but I often felt discouraged that so few people seemed upset by the fraudulent pretext for the war, now that Saddam was out of power. It was as if the entire nation was acting out the *Saturday Night Live* skit of Gilda Radner and Chevy Chase in which Gilda Radner goes on a long, mistaken rant and then suddenly declares, "Never mind."

If you pointed to the contradictions, most people would slough them off as no different than Bill Clinton lying about sex. Yet who in their right mind could equate lying about sex with lying to take a nation to war? It all seemed to confirm Morris Berman's assertion that the country had lost its intellectual discrimination and maybe its moral compass, as well.

Of course, there was another even darker possibility: that this was rooted in something much deeper—the banality of evil or the notion that fear and insecurity were germinating a fascist response. This is exactly the dynamic that Hannah Arendt had talked about in her cultural study of Nazi Germany. I shuddered at the thought that more Americans would soon be dying, as the enlightened warrior had predicted, and that this would usher in further violence and the erosion of civil liberties. The new Patriot Act proposed by Ashcroft was a chilling suggestion of that.

Civil Liberties in the Age of Ashcroft

First they came for the Communists, but I was not a Communist, so I said nothing. Then they came for the Social Democrats, but I was not a Social Democrat, so I did nothing. Then they came for the trade unionists, but I was not a trade unionist. And then they came for the Jews, but I was not a Jew, so I did little. Then when they came for me, there was no one left who could stand up for me.

Attributed to Pastor Martin Niemöller

Madeleine and I talked about these matters nearly every night, usually interspersed with a review of my health struggles. Sometimes the transitions between them were so seamless that they seemed one and the same: in mid-morning I awakened with an aching neck and brain fog and learned that a smoky veil was covering the Four Seasons in downtown Baghdad after a terrorist attack.

American gunships took to the air to support a Marine brigade that had moved in to pacify the area. Meanwhile I dropped four tabs of willow and reached for my electro-stimulation kit to zap the cervical spasms. By mid-morning the casualties were under treatment at a local hospital and I was able to catch a few hours of sleep.

Madeleine seemed concerned that I was wedded to a course of action that no longer seemed to be working. This was increasingly hard to deny. In early fall I suddenly began having severe back spasms. At first I thought these were caused by sleeping in the wrong position, but it soon became apparent that they weren't going away. In fact, they seemed to be spreading to my hips, rib cage, neck, and shoulders.

I knew I needed to try some new remedy, and I didn't mind lowering my standards of proof if I could find some relief. My acupuncturist said that I might want to try an exotic Chinese herbal concoction called Tung Shueh that was manufactured in Taiwan or Hong Kong and came in a box embossed with a hog's head. About ten years ago he had sold the stuff out of a broken-down pharmacy in LA's Chinatown. It worked miracles which he had witnessed first-hand. Chinamen would come to the pharmacy in wheelchairs or on crutches and return a few weeks later upright and healthy. Immediately I thought of Kwai Chang Caine working miracles with of his little brown pouch.

According to my acupuncturist, the ingredients were a little mysterious, but he was quite sure that they included dong quai root, pipefish, ding gong teng, and ginseng. Unfortunately, the original product was not readily available because of a bust by the FDA. Nevertheless I still might be able to find some in Chinatown. Short of that, I could probably find a less potent facsimile. He scribbled out an unpronounceable Chinese name and address and made me promise not to breathe a word to anyone.

In my best imitation of Jack Nicholson, I answered, "Jeezus man, who do you think you are dealing with?"

After two years of minimal travel and risk, except the occasional flyer on a longshot at Emerald Downs, drama had finally found its way to my doorstep. Not simply drama but intrigue—whispering, veiled, and forbidden intrigue that beckoned images of *Chinatown* starring Jack Nicholson. Chinatown was about going to a place where the normal rules no longer apply—a place of inscrutable mystery. People got lost in Chinatown and were never found. It was the underworld *nigredo* of Carl Jung, the Bedlam of Hieronymous Bosch, and the shadowland of Augustus Egg.

In the 1980s, I studied Chinatown from beginning to end and actually taught a class on it at Saint Mary's College in California. Yes, it was about time that Jake Gittes was back on the case. This time a much deeper conspiracy was brewing. It went beyond incest, beyond missing land deeds for orange groves in the Owens Valley, or the peculiar accounting in a rural rest home. The incriminating trail was littered with missing ballots from the Florida elections, seared letterhead telling of conversations between Dick Cheney and Ken DeLay, and transcripts that discussed the manipulation of oil prices and terrorist alerts before the Presidential elections. Maybe there were even deeper darker secrets to be excavated: why the networks had canceled *Kung Fu*, what had happened to George Bush's driving record, and why the American Rheumatism Association had tried so fervently to destroy Thomas McPherson Brown.

But I digress. The primary mission was to score some Tung Shueh and still the spasms in my aching back.

Under cover of early morning fog, Madeleine and I parked my rebuilt car on a Chinatown side-street and made our way north toward the Tao Lung Grocery, where my acupuncturist had told me to look for a Chinaman with a face that suggested shark fin soup. The aroma of fresh fish was in the air, the perfume of ginger and exotic Chinese herbs, and a sickly decay that I couldn't quite place. Perhaps it was the remains of someone who had said a little too much about a shady shipment of small brown balls coming in from Taiwan.

Madeleine wasn't traveling too well from her knee replacement, but I had to admit that she was cutting a fine form in her chic Faye Dunaway hat, choker necklace, and slinky rayon dress. If we got through this alive we would toast ourselves with martinis at an uptown gin joint.

I cast a gaze across the street and noticed a somewhat familiar looking organ grinder seated on an orange box dangling a puppet on strings. I just couldn't place the face. Then it came to me that he looked like a cop I often argued with about the illegitimacy of the war.

The resemblance was striking—same build, same jaded expression, same buzz-cutt. Only main difference was that this guy was wearing Al Franken glasses. Maybe I should queer the program by asking if he and his buddy George had come up with any concealed chemical weapons lately.

"Fuh'ged about it," counseled the Buddha who was trailing us in a fedora and trench coat and hanging a foul-smelling cigarette off the edge of his lip. He was right. In Chinatown, you minded your own business or you ended up feeding the pipefish in Hong Kong harbor.

We stumbled inside the Tao Lung grocery causing three elderly Chinese women working the registers to break out in a stream of Mandarin or whatever Chinese people spoke to hide their amusement about Anglos.

"What you need?" asked the head lady.

I decided to be discreet. "I'm looking for a fellow who knows something about a special herbal product."

I was about to try a different angle when a smirk appeared on her lips. "Danny," she cried out, "'nother customer need Tung Shueh big time."

Danny appeared behind a counter at the back of the store. When we arrived he dropped a small orange and magenta box on the counter. "Vine Essence," he declared. "Much like Tung Shueh; not quite as strong."

I inspected it closely. One panel was printed with strange hieroglyphics that looked like the magnified footprints of a cockroach. Another surface showed a visible man surrounded by a radiant yellow field, presumably resulting from the Vine

Essence. Another panel listed the ingredients. The print was very small and hard to read.

"It contains pipefish?"

"You betcha." He rattled off a list of Chinese herbs I had never heard of. "Sell five cases a week—sixty boxes. Everybody come back for more."

"How much per box?" I replied.

"Six dollar."

At first I didn't think I heard him correctly. The box alone was worth that.

"Five-fifty if you take a case," he blurted out.

"People buy it by the case?"

"Sometime supply get interrupted. No one want to be without."

I mulled it over for a full in-breath. "Gimme a case," I declared.

"You not regret it," he added.

Madeleine and I walked out of the store with a five-year supply of Tung Shueh.

The amazing thing was that it seemed to work. Within two days the pipefish, dong-quai root, and undisclosed exotica in those little brown balls somehow quelled my back spasms, soothed my inflammation, and spared me the unwanted drama of struggling to get out of bed in the morning.

Chapter 10

Journey on a Gurney to Bedlam

The mission to find the secret elixir in Chinatown provided a chance for both Madeleine and I to slip out of our skin, and for me to return to the unbounded drama of travel. The irony was that Seattle's Chinatown was only three miles from my apartment. It wasn't lost on me that during the entire episode I hadn't felt a single twinge of joint pain, one moment of dizziness, or twang of anxiety. Imagination had either eliminated all pain or simply masked it. It made me wonder whether this was simply a more elaborate form of acupuncture in which you brought your body to the needles rather than the other way around and the stimulus came from exotic aromas, sight, and sound jolting and energizing your *chi*.

The trip impressed on me just how extraordinary the ordinary could be. The only requirement was a dose of imagination and free-falling commitment. In daily routine, you so often miss the miraculous because reason and practical imperatives take over and it is difficult to get beyond the troubles the kids are having at school, the daily commuter grind, worries about finances, or perhaps controlling the inflammation in your aching joints.

One of the great tragedies of life-altering illness is that it can easily extinguish curiosity and play. You notice your world is shrinking and this causes further withdrawal. With each step backward you begin to encyst yourself behind a screen that admits no light and sound from the outside universe.

I saw this in my own father in the years after he contracted Parkinson's disease. The effect was insidious. He had always been an athlete and defined himself by what he did physically: how many miles he ran, how many holes of golf he played, how much grass he cut in our large frontyard and deposited in the city dump. The Parkinson's took away most of what he loved. His curiosity and interest in the world—vested mostly in sports and vigorous exercise—seemed to die. Even the sports page no longer held his interest.

Though my mother's illness was at least as painful as my father's, it didn't seem to extinquish her, but rather caused her to retreat to an inner sanctum. I had a pretty good idea what was going on there. For her, like so many other artists, reality was mutable and only limited by what she could envision. If she could imagine it, she could become at one with it in the same way that a soaring bird is at one with an updraft.

In a moment of intimate conversation several months before she fell ill, she confided in me that we shared a special kind of knowing that she had trouble talking about with others in her life. She reached for a book in which she had underlined a quote by the French painter Dubuffet. It described the experience of giving yourself up to a higher power when you painted. I knew that she felt the same way about music, dance, and acting.

Jean Dubuffet on Art

A picture interests me to the degree I succeed in kindling in it a kind of flame —the flame of life...To be sure, it often happens with me that my picture lacks this quality...In any case, I go on working, I add and I take away, I change, I revise until a certain extraordinary release occurs in the picture, and from then on it seems to me endowed with this very life—excuse me, reality. How can this be accounted for? I have no idea. I never know how I produced it, or how to repeat the same again effect.

Source: Jean Dubuffet, *Xxe Siecle* (quoted in *The Paintings of Henry Miller* by Henry Miller)

During the eleventh hour of her illness, she fell into a medicated sleep state much akin to a coma. At that point it was pretty clear that she wasn't going to survive. The doctors decided to bring her back to consciousness in a last-ditch attempt to save her. When she came to, her eyes were printed with disappointment. She had been jolted back to the invasive world of respirators, IVs, and the constant struggle with pain.

"Why would I have any interest in this?" she seemed to be pleading.

It was at this point that I knew that it would be a mistake to prolong her life.

When she finally died, I had a pretty good idea what happened to her soul. It immediately streaked for her home, which she never wanted to leave, despite the seriousness of her condition. Here she surely lingered over her paintings, tended to her beloved garden, and then, when she thought it was in order, levitated to the clouds.

In Dire Straits

Here she would have been reunited with Sky Carpenter, who himself had probably joined Vermeer, Albert Bierstadt, Rembrandt, and Van Gogh in reveling in the radiance of cirrus, cumulus, and cumulonimbus at sunset.

Madeleine and I both appreciated fantasy. For us the inner world was no less real than the outer. The physics were simply different. Our first conversation dated back to the early 1980s when she barged her way into a discussion I was having with a girlfriend about a movie. She had seen psychological layers to the film that I never would have imagined. From then on, we became close friends, frequently comparing notes on our favorite books.

I soon learned that she was one of the living experts on the writings of Henry Miller and Anais Nin. She had read everything by both of them and inspired me to read Miller on my own. His books and life story proved to be a great tonic for my writing.

At the time, I was struggling with a chaotic one thousand-page novel, my own version of *Portrait of an Artist*, but in this case it really was about an artist, a female, named Pierr Daumier. The story, entitled *Masters of Camouflage*, followed her upbringing on a houseboat in the Skagit River, where she was surrounded by radical and eccentric poets and painters.

Madeleine not only loved the story, but actually contributed to it with insights about family healing, the struggles of young girls to find an identity, and perils of being an orphaned child. Before long, I decided to write her into the story, along with her white shepherd, Penny.

The book gave Madeleine and I a creative vehicle to explore places and ideas. These included sorties into Impressionism, Gestalt Psychology, and the mysteries of camouflage. We also visited many of the places where major scenes occurred: the Skagit Marshland, the streets of Montparnasse, and the seedy alleys of Seattle's Skid Road.

By early 2000, the book was long since complete, and our repertory theatre largely revolved around our joint family of bears (including Schoomer and Big Sydney), as well as Buffy and the other dolls that my mom had passed on to us. We had incarnated them with fitting personalities. Schoomer was the ultimate trickster and harlequin, always at his best on Halloween; Big Sydney was the consummate healer; and Buffy showed no interest whatsoever in Buddha nature and contented herself with singing, dancing, and stuffing herself with chocolate.

By fall of 2002, they had all taken on a mischievous vitality that neither Madeleine nor I could control. Suddenly they were scheming to see who could come up with the best Halloween costume. When the competition was over, Buffy prevailed as an oversized Queen Bee (clad in a velvet bee suit complete with menacing yellow antennae); Schoomer finished a close second as a psychedelic swami in a multi-colored wig that would have envied Don King; and Big Sydney wowed the other dolls and bears as an energy healer, complete with Groucho Marx nose glasses, stethoscope, and healing pyramid.

Both of us needed as much comic relief as possible to deal with the daily news from Iraq. In early fall of 2003, propagandists for the administration were claiming that the war was defensible because Saddam the butcher, gasser, and shredder, had been removed. The spiel usually included an implied link between Saddam and the 9/11 attacks. If ever there was a verbal counterpart to camouflage and the techniques of Abbott Thayer and M.C. Escher, it was this.

The original camoufleurs explored the ways animals were confused by or took advantage of shade and dazzling colors. A gazelle, for example, was hard to detect at a distance because her undersides were brighter than her torso, which is just the opposite of what you would expect under normal overhead sunlight. This was called countershading.

Mimicry was another favored technique of animals in the wild. Poisonous snakes often displayed a sequence of colored rings that reflected the old saw—red after yellow will kill a fellow. But many non-poisonous snakes mimicked them with red rings followed by black ones. The charade was convincing enough to scare away possible predators.

Escher took perceptual trickery to a higher level with mind traps showing how easily the eye could be confused by the seemingly logical. His specialty was the confusion of figure and ground. One of the best examples was *Ascending and Descending March* that pictured several faceless drudges trapped in a staircase that simultaneously ascended and descended. The only way to escape the staircase was to step out of it—to refuse to accept its seductive illogic.

The charades of Karl Rove, Fox News, and "Neo-Con" radio talk shows still seemed to be holding up. One of their latest techniques was to ask whether you were safer or better off without Saddam Hussein? I recognized this immediately:

they were trying to enforce the perverse rules of the staircase: drudges were only allowed to place one foot after the other. The past, particularly that period during which the staircase was being designed and built, was out of bounds.

Whenever Howard Dean, Dennis Kucinich, or a like-minded critic harkened back to the reasons for the invasion, the Administration and their media connections fired back that these people were caught up in the past. When someone posed the question about Saddam to Ray McGovern, Joseph Wilson, and the best of the war critics, they violated staircase rules and challenged the architecture of the staircase: Are we better off? All things considered? No, we are worse off. We have alienated much of the Muslim world, vastly increased the pool of terrorist recruits, and antagonized our allies. Beyond that, we have short-shrifted our troops in Afghanistan, created a monumental debt that has weakened our economy, and maybe worst of all, have forfeited the moral high ground by going to war on the basis of a lie.

In September 2003, even my daily writing about Bush propaganda supporting the Iraq invasion couldn't mask the fact that the Chinese elixir was no longer working. The pain had returned and was erupting across my back. My greatest fear was that the disease might be attacking my kidneys because this was where the pain seemed to be centered. I scheduled an appointment with my primary care doctor, hoping that she could provide help or at least diagnose what was going on. In short order she ruled out kidney problems. She wasn't exactly sure what was going on, only that muscles, tendons, and ligaments were inflamed.

In Dire Straits

My relief over the condition of my kidneys gave way to the realization that I was now suffering from spondylitis. This only seemed to occur in the most extreme renditions of psoriatic arthritis. I hated to think where this would lead if I didn't do something. I didn't need to wait very long to find out because only a few days later, spasms erupted all along my spine and rib cage, causing discomfort from breathing and making it virtually impossible to walk.

Madeleine kept prodding me to tell her what my plan was. My reply was usually terse and defensive: "Stick with the plan."

Finally she provoked a stream of discouragement: "Look, I've tried steroids; I've tried diet; I've tried herbs; I've tried everything I can think of to amplify the effects of the antibiotics. Maybe I'll just roll up in a tight ball."

"I didn't realize you thought it was hopeless."

The comment stopped me dead in my tracks. Was this what I was saying?

"Exactly what you are saying," declared the Buddha. "What a sniveling weenie you are."

In early November, after a few days of relief, I awakened on a Monday morning with acute chest pain. I didn't think it was a heart attack, but was in such discomfort that I needed help immediately. I called Madeleine and she suggested I go to the fire station a few blocks from my apartment. There I could ask the firemen to check my heart and blood pressure. If I needed emergency help, they could send for an ambulance to take me to the hospital.

When I arrived at the station, an EMT was summoned to

assess my condition. As he checked my vital signs, he interrogated me about my symptoms: did I feel any shortness of breath or numbness in my extremities? No, none at all.

I explained that I had many joint and muscle pains from my arthritis, and of late they had migrated to my rib cage. Perhaps this was more of the same. He seemed unconvinced. He scanned the screen of his portable EKG machine and declared to one of the hovering firemen that the results were "uncertain." What exactly did that mean? He gave me an aspirin and reached for a radio to speak to an emergency room doctor at Virginia Mason Hospital.

I couldn't quite make out the response, but apparently it wasn't that positive because several firemen began helping me onto a gurney. We were headed for the hospital. I sighed heavily. It was probably a good idea to see a doctor, even if I was just having muscle problems.

As the ambulance alarm began to shriek and the van began snaking through traffic, the medic placed a tab of nitroglycerin under my tongue. Suddenly the seriousness of my situation dawned on me. You didn't give someone nitroglycerin for no reason at all. Maybe I hadn't yet had an attack but was on the verge of one. Did my heart feel as though it was about about to explode? Not really.

The medic asked if I felt any better and I said that I could still feel spasms and pain but the sensation was more like a deep ache than a spike. Suddenly he seemed more concerned. Did I say the wrong thing? He placed an oxygen tube up my nose and again reached for the radio. Apparently the doctor was concerned that the nitro hadn't helped and wanted me to take a second tab.

The medic started to place another under my tongue but I decided to speak out: "Are you sure this is a good idea?"

"The doc says so and he's the boss." Reluctantly I let him place it in my mouth. Only a few minutes later the world started moving entirely too fast. We reached the emergency bay at the hospital and before I could really orient myself, several people were lifting the gurney and then wheeling me through a double doorway down a wide, overly bright corridor.

Lying there flat on my back, I felt the sensation of riding a small boat down a turbulent river. I remembered a similar sensation in traveling down the Moselle River in 1996. The river was deeply incised within valley walls and you got used to looking high up on the ridge at a succession of medieval ramparts and parapets. In the process, you missed the fact that the river was teeming with barges and riverboats streaming at you lickitty-split. We scraped against a gurney to my right and then left.

Out of the corner of my eye I caught a glimpse of the unfortunate patients. They were in their eighties, frail and abject. In the Middle Ages, lost souls from the burgs of Northern Europe were commonly relegated to barges on the Rhine. Bosch and Brant depicted this in their artwork.

A stream of arcane medical-speak was filling the air— something about proximeters and a speculum, or more likely the tools of a chymist licensed in the black art of rheumatology? And then some kind of buzzer began sounding up ahead. We came closer to the room and a shriek filled the air. "Please, someone help me. Please." It was the forlorn cry of Bedlam, the kind of orphaned fright that would have inspired Edvard Munch or Hans Belmer. What exactly had I signed up for? We clipped another gurney and managed to remain on the thalweg while passing a bobbing fleet of other helpless souls, unattended by staff.

Some time around 1550, Hieronymous Bosch created *Ship of Fools* that externalized the darkest, sordid forces in the human psyche. The ship was really a prow, not much larger from bow to stern than my gurney, and packed with lost souls. A particularly fearful sot was cowering in the stern, next to a kind-looking nun in a white scarf who had placed her hand on his shoulder. Yet, her own intentions weren't exactly clear. If you looked closely, you could see that she seemed to be nudging him toward a liquid dripping from an overhead urn. Perhaps it was the elixir of knowledge, but it could also have been hemlock. All was open to interpretation in the bizarre underworld of Bosch.

I really wished I hadn't taken that extra tab of nitro. You really wanted to be in full command of your senses if you were floating toward Bedlam in a small unseaworthy boat.

An image came to me of my mom in her last month. She was at home after a round of chemo. She had fallen sick and the doctors insisted that she return to the hospital. She pleaded with me not to take her to the emergency room for fear that she wouldn't return. If her time had come, she wanted to die at home surrounded by her garden and all that she loved.

I tried to explain to her that she needed help and only a doctor could provide it. I tried to reassure her that she would be OK, and that as soon as she got over the setback she could return home. She only curled up in a tight ball. An hour later, after much coaxing, she relented but a look of bewildered surrender glazed her eyes as we carried her to the car. I guess I didn't realize what she understood instinctively—that this would be a trip from which she wouldn't return.

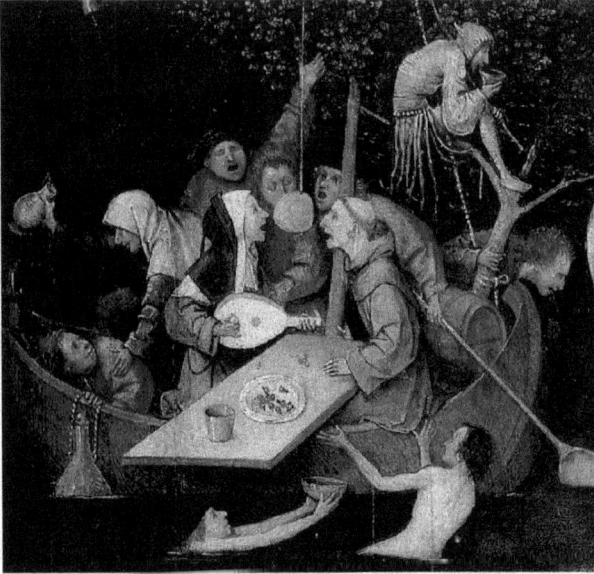

Source: Louvre, Paris, France

Was I capable of pulling myself up, releasing the strap, and jumping ship before the cliff drop? The straps didn't seem that tight. They were almost free when a burst of pain threw me back against my pillow. I really did need to see a doctor.

The gurney floated forward through the hallway, and just when I thought we might be passing through another set of double doors, we steered to the left and into a treatment room. All I could see were several disembodied faces that seemed alert and animate, maybe a little speedy. A nurse inserted a catheter into my arm and said something about an IV and I made no protest. Another fellow, apparently the head doctor, drew close and wanted to know how I was feeling. Maybe only to regain some control, I said, "I think I'm doing OK. Really. Just a bit dizzy at the moment...About the heart pain—I think it's related to my psoriatic arthritis."

"We're going to check you out completely, to find out exactly what is going on here." A nurse began attaching leads to my chest, presumably for more monitoring. Another nurse drew blood for a test that would determine the presence of enzymes released from a heart attack.

I thought I recognized the head doctor from my days playing basketball. Yes, I was now sure of it. We had even checked each other. He was methodical and heady, a good team player, but not very offensive-minded. I suppose those weren't bad qualities in a doctor. Did he recognize me as well? If so, I hoped I hadn't fouled him too badly. People remembered that sort of thing.

He reached for a stethoscope, and after listening to my heartbeat asked what I did for a living.

"I guess my main occupation is writing," I answered with a grimace from another spasm.

"Oh really, and what do you write about?" he answered moving on to my reflexes.

I sighed. "Well of late, I've been doing everything in my power to reveal the phony pretext for this unconstitutional war in Iraq."

This seemed to get the attention of everyone in the room

and it occurred to me that I had a captive audience. "I figured somebody had to stand up and confront the nonsense."

My doctor chuckled and then retreated through the doorway to help on another procedure.

A few minutes later he returned, and after declaring that my EKG was normalizing added, "What was the name of the pub that you won at the racetrack?"

"What?"

"I looked you up on the web and read the back cover of one of your books. It said that you won a pub by making an outrageous horse bet."

Now everyone wanted to hear the story, so I gave them the abridged version: "With two other friends I tried to open an Irish pub near Seattle but we ran out of money." I drew a deep breath. "We took all that we had left and sent it on a longshot at the races—a very gutsy filly that my partner helped raise. We got lucky. She won in a photo finish."

Everyone seemed to enjoy the story and pressed for more details: how close was the photo? How much did win? Did we celebrate?"

"Celebrated like drunken sailors."

My glory was interrupted by the head doctor declaring that because of limited space he had to move me to a holding area. He didn't think that I had had a heart attack, but wouldn't know for sure until my blood tests were processed.

I nodded and he asked whether my pain was tolerable.

"I can handle it," I answered.

I felt much relieved by the news, but was probably more buoyed by the fact that he liked my story.

"You really are an egotistical fool," came an uninvited voice behind me. It was my cherubic Buddhist roommate. It had never occurred to me that he had come along for the ride.

"Always like a good cruise down the river," he declared. "You realize that I worked as a ferryman in India?"

"Yes, we've heard that story before, my friend." I had to admit it was good to have him at my side. I would let him handle the gurney since he professed to be such an experienced boatman.

The Ferryman and the River

I will remain by this river, thought Siddhartha. It is the same river which I crossed on my way to the town. A friendly ferryman took me across... (Siddhartha) looked lovingly into the flowing water, into the transparent green, into the crystal lines of its wonderful design. He saw bright pearls rise from the depths, bubbles swimming on the mirror, sky blue relected in them. The river looked at him with a thousand eyes—green, white, crystal, sky blue. How he loved this river, how it enchanted him, how grateful he was to it! In his heart he heard the newly awakened voice speak, and it said to him: "love this river, stay by it, learn from it."

Source: Herman Hesse, *Siddhartha*

The first results were negative but not conclusive, so I had to take another test and wait for the report. Several times over the next hour, the aches and spasms erupted, but each time I was able to soften them with deep breathing and other relaxation techniques I had learned from Steven Levine.

"I'm going to get through this," I would murmur. And then the Buddha would add, "Watch breath, soften belly, open heart. Piece of cake."

In Dire Straits

In moments of calm, I found myself observing the barge traffic on the river. First came a wave of trauma resulting from a multiple car-accident. The less important barges, including my own, were pressed against the bank, and the channel was filled with nurses and doctors rushing by with IVs and floating new equipment into place. Less than an hour later, the frantic activity ended and I wasn't exactly sure why. Perhaps the trauma had been carried downstream, beyond those double doors at the end of the hall to even more turbulent waters, perhaps patrolled by much more serious ferrymen clad in black scrubs.

Then a calm descended, and I could almost hear the water lapping against the bank—so very quiet and still—and if you gazed into a pool you could see bubbles rising to the surface, each one containing a recognizable face from the past. In each bubble a tiny theatre seemed to be playing out, complete with the sound of my own voice in conversation—resistant, willful, and idealistic. I was really too unaccepting to be a very good Buddhist—too much into remaking the world on my own terms. I guess this was why art and literature held such appeal. You could create whatever world you wanted to live in.

Madeleine arrived and broke my reverie. She asked what she could do to help. I told her that I was doing fine, but needed to use the lavatory. She unloosened the gurney straps and I started down the hallway with my IV bag. After only a few steps I began to teeter. I tried to compensate, but couldn't find a balance point. Madeleine caught me just as I started to fall. I was very lucky to have someone like her watching over me.

My doctor was waiting for me when I returned. "No heart attack," he declared cheerfully. "You're free to go if you feel strong enough." Madeleine mentioned my near-fall, and he suggested that I might want to wait until I became steadier. As for the heart pains and spasms, he could offer no explanation, but was sure that they were not life-threatening.

Within an hour my equilibrium returned and Madeleine escorted me to the main door of the emergency room. I was no sooner outside than a piercing cold shivered my bones. It was a mild forty-five degrees outside, but I felt like a sailor overboard in the North Atlantic. Apparently the nitro had dilated my pores. My teeth began to chatter and I wondered if I could actually make it to the car. The last hundred yards were a desperate lunge.

Coherent speech eluded me the entire ride home. When I reached my apartment, I streaked for my bed and buried myself under a mountain of blankets. Schoomer and Big Sydney piled on top to keep me warm.

A few days later, my heartaches lessened and I began to reflect on the experience. Nietzsche had said, "If you stare into the abyss, it will stare back at you." In some sense this is what happened. The abyss aroused my curiosity and so too the current before the falls. Instead of letting my anxiety get the better of me and clinging to the side of the prow, I braved a few looks over the side and was surprised by what I found. It wasn't as terrifying as I imagined. Certainly there were more than a few good ferrymen working the river, helping the frail and disabled with the difficulties of passage.

In Dire Straits

140

Chapter 11

Ruminations Under the Drip

A few days after I returned from the hospital, I learned that Ralph had located a doctor friend in the Midwest who recommended an IV protocol that included doxycycline, DMSO, and several natural anti-inflammatories. It wasn't based upon any overarching theory or critically evaluated research, but medical empiricism, that bastard stepchild to hard science, expressing the idea that if something works, it probably merits trying again under reasonably similar circumstances and maybe fiddling with it to amplify effectiveness.

For five days straight I visited Ralph's office, and while his empirical cocktail seeped into my blood, I reflected on my deteriorating condition, usually while scanning a book on healing or an allied topic. It had now been three years from the onset of my condition. Throughout the ordeal I had tried to be thorough and rational in researching the disease and the possible treatments. In the process, I had focused mostly on physiological remedies rather than the spiritual ones. So far I had refrained from smoking ayahuasca with a Yaqui shaman, avoided toothy fundamentalists with one hand on your forehead and the other on your wallet, and steered clear of psychic healers promising to extract a toxic frog from your crown chakra.

I had to admit that I found some of the ideas appealing —at least from an artistic point of view. But so far I had enforced a firm limit on my medical practice of Dada. When it came to immune system function, heart, kidney, lungs, and digestion, I was decidedly a rationalist. Then, too, vanity and self-image prevented me from experiments that were too radical. I wasn't ready to look like a mindless flake just to get better. Maybe this was my limitation.

On my first IV, Ralph noticed that I was reading a book by Dr. Larry Dossey, the well-known author on the spiritual side of healing. He said they had met at a conference, and I replied with an observation by Dossey about the uncertainty in so much medicine—"Sometimes there is only a cloud of unknowing and the best you can do is stand in the mystery." It was an allusion to the fourteenth-century Christian treatise about the mysterious workings of grace and the fact that patients sometimes had no option other than to leave their fate to a higher power. Ralph smiled. I wasn't sure if he agreed or just liked the metaphor.

Until the onset of my disease, I probably accorded more sophistication and rigor to medicine than it deserved. It came as shock to discover how little was really known about most rheumatological disease—Doctor Brown had made the persuasive case. The profession couldn't even decide whether most of one hundred-some rheumatoid disorders were variations on a single disease. Their support for steroids and methotrexate was completely baffling because it wasn't based on proven efficacy.

When it came to the role of thought and emotion and how they affected biochemistry, you were deep into the clouds. Researchers in the new field of psychoneuroimmunology were exploring some of the more bounded issues while a smaller group of scientists were speculating on the effects of consciousness on energy and the ramifications to cell and organ function. Researchers giving this much attention usually raised eyebrows and became candidates for a three-sided hat and a sanitorium jumpsuit.

But there were at least a few who managed to avoid the label of jester or charlatan, Dossey among them. My list also included Herbert Benson, Bernie Siegel, Dean Ornish, and Candace Pert. Other writers I wasn't ready to dismiss out-of-hand included Gary Zukav, Amit Goswami, Michael Talbot, W. Brugh Joy, Deepak Chopra, Jean Achtenberg, Bruce Lipton, Barbara Brennan, Carolyn Myss, and Stanislav Grof.

Ralph usually checked in on me every ten minutes, and when he did I would treat him to the latest firing of neurons across my brain. It might be another dose of Dossey or my own hybrid links between the Heisenberg Uncertainty Principle and over-active T-cells. Sometimes the look on his face suggested that he thought he had given me the wrong medication. On other occasions I could tell he wanted to reply but knew his patient load wouldn't permit it. I didn't mind his reticence. I was mostly verbalizing for myself—examining what I believed and what I might be missing that could arrest the decline in my health. Maybe if that failed, I could still discover a way to cope with it. The experience at the hospital had lessened some of my more irrational fears about medicine but it had also awakened me to the possibility that this might be a disease that I didn't fully recover from.

In *Recovering the Soul*, Larry Dossey constructed a bridge between healing and quantum mechanics. Citing the arguments and speculation of David Bohm, Edwin Schrodinger, as well as several theoretical biologists, he made the case that the human mind, at least occasionally, organizes and creates in a way that transcends normal time/space limitations. He was clearly interested in the deeper layers of the clouds and maybe the implicate order wherein thought was energized and transformed to matter.

His books offered many examples of quantum healing in which patients seemed to achieve an energetic, psychokinetic communion with a higher or collective intelligence. (Much of the research had been done by the Institute for Noetic Studies, founded by the astronaut, Edgar Mitchell.) Apparently most spontaneous cures occurred among patients who were open and accepting and not particularly desperate for a remission. Many also displayed a distant gaze, suggesting that they might have altered their own consciousness.

I recalled that Michael Murphy at Esalen and the author of *The Future of the Body* had compiled a list of various extraordinary physical, mental, and spiritual phenomena. His inquiry included telekinesis, artistic inspiration, psychokinesis (PK), remarkable performances in sports, and the feats of Hindu yogis. A case could be made that spontaneous remissions and the other PK events were related. In each case, a person seemed to be tapping a non-local power.

Dossey, Amit Goswami, Fred Allen Wolf, Michael Talbot, and Rupert Sheldrake made much of non-locality. Certainly at the sub-atomic level, thought and energy displayed interconnectedness at a distance (non-locality), which transcended Newtonian mechanics and even the notions of relativity advanced by Einstein. Rupert Sheldrake had done some of the most interesting work in this area, positing the existence of morphic fields that were created by repetitive behavior. This was consistent with the ideas of the physicist, David Bohm, who speculated on the existence of an implicate order beyond the material world that could affect matter and organize it functionally.

Of course, the local effects of relaxation were hardly trivial, and for the most part, accepted by conventional medicine. Dr. Herbert Benson in *The Relaxation Response* actually demonstrated that relaxation decreased metabolism, blood pressure, heart rate, rate of breathing, and muscle tension. A wealth of data also supported the benefits of love, joy, and laughter to the immune system, including the production of Immunoglobulin A, the body's first defense against colds and other viral diseases. Most researchers saw no need to ascribe this to non-locality.

But Dossey and others were clearly talking about something more—a quantum event in which a person could channel and mobilize healing energy from the collective unconscious, a divinity, or higher power. Their stories of miraculous healing were so unusual and beyond daily experience that they seemed dubious, but many were hard to refute. The story of the Jansenist "convulsionaries" described by Michael Talbot in *The Holographic Universe* was especially compelling.

It seems that in 1727, a sect of Dutch-influenced Catholics known as Jansenists gained popularity with the French masses because of a charismatic leader, Francois de Paris, and the fact that members of the order seemed able to perform miracle cures.

By venturing into the domain of miracles, the Jansenists provoked serious concern in Rome. Church insiders were already troubled by the irredentist tendencies of the Jansenists. Some even considered them Protestants in disguise. But the issue was not simply accounting for the anomalous events but maintaining Church monopoly or at least authority over mystical phenomena. As both Michael Murphy and Morris Berman have described, miracles, the workings of "grace," and divine intervention lie at the core of Catholic canon and date back to the formation of the Church. In fact, protecting authority was a primary (though not exclusive) motivation of the Church in its efforts to do away with the Albigensians in Gaul in the thirteenth Century A.D. No doubt the Church hadn't forgotten that apostasy and were suspicious that the Jansenists were brewing up something similar.

During one of my IVs, I read that on May 1, 1727, the incipient heresy took a strange turn after the death of Francois. In Paris, his worshippers and mourners gathered at his tomb and began to perform healings of cancer, blindness, paralysis, arthritis, and rheumatism. Among the cured was the niece of the mathematician and philosopher Pascal. Apparently a severe ulcer was removed from her eye.

A bizarre aspect of the healings was that they started with unafflicted priests and laity who suddenly began to experience involuntary convulsions. Seemingly possessed, these people would circulate among the crowd, healing the sick and simultaneously displaying the most phenomenal physical abilities, including feats of bizarre strength, demonstrations of clairvoyance, and invulnerability to abuse. Apparently, true-believers showed no ill effects after being crucified, struck with thirty-pound hammers, stabbed, and choked.

The incidents weren't simply isolated, but occurred in the open over a several year period during which they were widely observed by both scholars and Church emissaries. One of those dispatched to investigate was Louis Basile Carre de Montgeron, a member of the Paris Parliament. His findings filled four volumes. He reported that the miracles were so numerous that three thousand volunteers were engaged to assist the convulsionaries, "and make sure, for example, that the female participants did not become immodestly exposed during their seizures."

The image of the mass exposure came to me during my IV just as Ralph was checking my progress. "Damn! That must have been a sight."

Ralph shot me a curious look and headed off to attend to another patient. I would have to fill him in later on my travel experiences in France and my enduring love of sexy Parisian women.

In Dire Straits

By my estimation, most writers on PK events believed that the elimination of fear (and fear-based emotions) was the best explanation for the various phenomena. It was as if the cosmos were constantly bombarding humankind with miraculous possibilities and anyone could receive them as long as their tuner weren't draped in a lead X-ray blanket.

The more I reflected on this, the less convinced I was. Artistic inspiration, also a PK phenomenon in my mind, required more than openness. You had to do much more than eliminate the lead shield on the tuner. You had to be able to set the dials. And of course, no one was going to receive a decent signal unless they had high-fidelity equipment. This was a critical mistake in most new-age theory—the assumption that everyone was innately gifted.

Gary Zukav, one of my favorite writers, offered a related version of mind over matter in *Seat of the Soul.* In his view, the body was the instrument of the soul and people were spiritual beings manifested in a body. Taking this one step further, he suggested that disease tends to reflect the state of the soul and struggles a person is having with personal meaning. There seemed to be three important issues that he was merging together: the ability of mindset to create disease; the role of mindset in determining a specific manifestation; and the curative power of spiritual practice. Without some pretty strong evidence, I certainly wasn't going to buy the idea that a dis-eased spirit caused all or most illness or that failure to heal necessarily reflected some spiritual inadequacy.

I guess I sided with Ken and Treya Wilber on this. In *Grace and Grit* they argued that the etiology of most disease was simply too complex to claim that mindset was the main or critical determinant of healing. Genetics came into play as well as environmental influences; so, too, nutrition and certainly chance (especially if you included accidents).

The Effect of Mind on Disease

One's emotional, mental, and spiritual makeup can most definitely influence physical illness and physical healing, just as a physical illness can have strong repercussions on the higher levels...The question, then is just how much downward causation does the mind—do our thoughts and emotions—have on physical illness? And the answer seems to be: much more than was once thought, not nearly as much as new-agers believe.

Source: Ken Wilber, *Grace and Grit*

The Wilber's also had direct experience of their own. Treya, Ken's wife, contracted breast cancer soon after they were married. She was a most gentle, conscious, and loving person, with a disciplined spiritual practice. If anyone was a candidate for remission it was Treya Wilber, but she died after a long and difficult struggle in which she displayed uncommon determination and equanimity.

In re-reading this gripping story, I was convinced that Treya's death could not have been avoided through any spiritual practice. Her cancer, as Ken described, was one of the Nazis of the microbiological world. No amount of loving kindness gratitude or mindfully projected *ahimsa* was going to win it over to non-violence.

On occasion during my IVs, I would be visited by Ralph's dog Bella, a sweet brown lab with an interesting healing story of her own that was related to me by Ralph's wife and office manager, Charlyn. According to Charlyn, about a year back, Bella awakened one morning and could only use her back legs. Within an hour she was paralyzed and could only crawl to get around.

Charlyn took her to the vet and learned that she was suffering from a fibro-cartilaginous embolism—a relative rare disorder that most commonly affects athletes, both canine and human, who have been subjected to severe back stress. Charlyn added that ever since Bella was a puppy, Bella had been an extraordinary Frisbee fetcher, jumper, and ball-retriever.

The vet admitted her to the animal hospital, but after three days Bella didn't respond to treatment and the vet advised the Golans that the situation was bleak: the embolism had apparently done permanent damage to her spinal cord. Ralph and Charlyn took her home but weren't yet ready to put her down. On a daily basis they carried her in a sling to the front yard so that she would have a chance to be with them in the sunshine. Bella had always been an outdoor dog.

On one of these occasions, Ralph actually gave her a high-potency vitamin IV and Bella remained still and calm all through the procedure. But as soon as it was over, she began crawling for the garden. Charlyn found this most unusual. Bella was never the sort of dog that dug up plants and rolled in the dirt, but now she seemed obsessed with it. Charlyn scolded her but it didn't seem to do any good. Bella just wanted to get back to the dirt. Ralph and Charlyn now feared the worst—that the embolism was also causing dementia.

Figuring they were running out of options, Charlyn

decided to take Bella to a Chinese acupuncturist much experienced in treating animals. The woman took Bella's pulses and set about mixing a Chinese herbal concoction she was certain would help. When it was ready, Charlyn removed the cap and took a whiff. The stench was so bad it practically knocked her over. She was sure Bella wouldn't touch it. The acupuncturist suggested mixing it with her food. Charlyn agreed to give it a try but remained skeptical. On the way out Charlyn asked what was in the concoction and the acupuncturist replied that the main constituent was earthworm.

For Charlyn, rockets fired and whistles sounded: Bella had been rooting through the garden—was it possible that she was looking for earthworms to heal herself? The acupuncturist had no opinion on Bella's instincts but advised that she would be fine if she took the medicine regularly for two months.

Bella devoured the earthworm pate with relish and within three days was up and wobbling around on all fours. Within a week she was frolicking like a puppy. At first chance she bolted into the front yard, but strangely enough, showed no interest in the garden. She only wanted to race circles around Ralph and Charlyn and retrieve Frisbees. Days later, she still showed no interest in the dirt.

After a month Charlyn and Bella returned to the acupuncturist for a follow-up appointment. The woman took Bella's pulses and prescribed another concoction, this time containing no earthworm. Apparently Bella no longer suffered from that deficiency.

The story accented my belief that all creatures are not endowed equally. Sheldrake discusses this in *Dogs That Know*

When Their Owners Are Coming Home. The book details the uncanny ability of many pets to read their owner's intentions. Some are so perceptive that they can detect the onset of epilepsy or heart attacks. Still other pets are impressively imperceptive, possibly because of domestication or simply individual differences. I was quite sure that Bella belonged among the adepts of her breed, among the canine counterparts to the Shaolin masters. When I asked Ralph and Charlyn about this, they confirmed it: she always seemed to know when they were headed home and could read their intentions.

As I write these words, I am still in the process of winning over Bella to my healing team. I figure that if I can create the proper bond, perhaps with a few favored dog biscuits, I can motivate her to go rooting for me in the garden and come up with just the right herb, mushroom, or earthworm to modulate my immune system and get rid of the bugs.

Chapter 12

Dirt Management and Dada

I couldn't stop thinking about Bella's healing story. I was sure that I would have concluded as Charlyn did that Bella was struggling to get to the garden because she was sick and losing her mind. It never would have dawned on me that she was following some kind of inner knowing or instinct.

A few weeks after hearing the story, I found discussion of "the problem of dirt" in Daniel Goleman's *Vital Lies, Simple Truths*. Goleman used different terms, but was addressing the same basic issue—making sense of unsorted facts and accounting for anomaly. He made much of the fact that all frames possessed blindspots and inherently oversimplified. When something didn't fit, the normal response was to deny the contrary evidence as either false or irrelevant—essentially to sweep it under the rug, rather than question and maybe change the frame.

The war in Iraq seemed to be a perfect example. As long as it was clean and costless, people were willing to accept the phony pretext for the war and all the fear-laden propaganda to sell it. Only when the dead American bodies began to accumulate did this change. Now, people were raising questions about everything from the missing WMD to the strange events at Abu Ghraib Prison. The Bush Administration clearly had a dirt management problem on its hands and the inconvenient dust was turning into a mountain of slag. If they didn't soon get this under control, all credibility would be lost and maybe sweep their party out of power in the 2004 elections.

I wondered about my own frame and convenient self-assurances. Even though I had survived the ordeal at Virginia Mason hospital, was I really getting any better? Was I performing a glorious dirt-sweep of my own? The problem for me was that it was so darn hard to separate symptoms from Herxheimer (or die-off) that supposedly indicated that you were killing bacteria and healing. In both cases you experienced inflammation, which might come in the form of dizziness, joint soreness, and a variety of other neurological symptoms. So many of these were also symptoms of the disease.

According to Dr. Brown, you could often differentiate the two. Supposedly a herx came a few days after a round of antibiotics; supposedly it was short-lived. Trouble was, reality wasn't so neat. Some inflammation came immediately before or after taking antibiotics, but even that might not quickly pass. It was always a guessing game to figure out exactly what was going on. Then, of course, there was the mystery of what had caused my heart palpitations and sent me to emergency room. Was that also caused by die-off and a release of toxins?

In a book about Camouflage Art, I discovered that Dada

was also involved in dirt management, or to be more apt—manure spreading. The intent was to skewer, lampoon, demythologize, and disrobe empty values by spreading and celebrating them. Their target was bourgeois society, crass commercialism, corrupt, hypocritical religion, and nationalism.

Marcel Duchamp gave the Mona Lisa a mustache and goatee; George Grosz cast businessmen as automatons and ciphers; and Max Ernst mustered the unmitigated gall to create a frottage entitled, *Virgin Spanking the Infant Jesus (1926)*.

Defenders of the order accused the avant-garde of hating society, but that itself was a distortion. Actually they appreciated the dazzling leaps of imagination reflected in symbols and myth. Their problem was with the underlying values and particularly how people allowed themselves to be manipulated into supporting wars of empire and to give up their own freedom and individuality.

Cheese and the Universe

The universe would appear to be something like a cheese; it can be sliced in an infinite number of was—and when one has chosen his own pattern of slicing, he finds that other men's cuts fall at the wrong places.

Source: Kenneth Burke, *Permanence and Change*

It wasn't lost on me that my attitude about treatment was significantly affected by the trauma of my mom's death. I felt she had been railroaded into taking toxic drugs that left her dependent on nurses and doctors. This was something doctors never explained: once you agreed to chemotherapy, at the slightest hint of a cold you had to be ready to return to the hospital. Therapy was also adjusted constantly to account for side effects.

There were other dirty little secrets and deceits, not the least of which was the scandal that a huge number of people died annually while in the hospital from drug-resistant staph bacteria. That's what eventually killed my mom.

Despite the deceit and lack of full disclosure, I knew that a blanket condemnation would be an overreaction. My mom might still have died and suffered just as much if she had turned down chemotherapy. My gripe, I suppose, was that she was rushed to choose and then not given full information.

I found an interesting book on Dada and Surrealism that gave special attention to belief and behavior grounded on fear and panic. My favorite example was Max Ernst's *Two Children Are Menaced by a Nightengale (1926)*. It actually depicted a young girl fleeing in mortal terror from a nightingale. If you looked closely you could see that the painting even included a red panic button that the viewer could press to summon help. The brilliance of the image was that it rattled your own frame: it provoked you to think about your own panic buttons, fearful associations, and how you acted on them.

In another art book I discovered that when Surrealism blossomed in the late 1920s, a shift occurred. Art became less scatological with more focus on dreamland and the subconscious—also the unstable boundary between reality and reverie.

Dreamscapes abounded, some of them whimsical but often with a disquieting twist. Salvador Dali's *Persistence of Memory* was one of the best examples, and so too, Rene

Magritte's several depictions of the human condition (1933–1935). Whether they realized it or not, Dali, Magritte, and Ernst were trespassing into quantum territory, wherein all forms were transmutable and spontaneously shifted between matter and energy.

But they weren't simply innocent explorers. Anarchy and revolt were on the agenda and along with Hans Bellmer, Georgio de Chirico, Alberto Giacometti, and Luis Bunuel, they gathered shovels and pales and headed into the darkest parts of the garden to root out the juiciest night crawlers and spread the rot. Their more visceral and upsetting contributions included *Woman with Her Throat Cut* (Giacometti, 1932) and *The Butterflies Begin to Sing* (Ernst 1929).

In thinking about this, I wondered what Max Ernst or filmmaker Luis Bunuel would have made of the climate of fear in the United States since 9/11. They would have to be impressed by the Manichean skill of Bush in defining friend and foe, and skillfully linking the Sodomite of Baghdad to the smoking trade towers; also, the less-than-subtle suggestions that he, George Bush, was on a mission from God to smite the evil-doers. Ernst, especially, would have loved the manipulation of the terror alerts.

In the 1920s, Bunuel produced two shocking and somewhat revolting commentaries on the rise of fascism, *L'age d'or* and *Un Chien Andelou*. The latter cast a dog in a key role. Bunuel, I was confident, would have immediately recognized Bella's special gifts and starred her in an update of *Un Chien*.

I had a pretty good idea how the film would play out. It would begin with Bella rooting through the garden on all fours, feverishly churning up worms. The soundtrack would offer chastising cries from Ralph and Charlyn, plus an overdubbing of the panic in New York on 9/11.

The action would cut to George Bush in flight suit appealing to the masses to join the posse. His Texas drawl would be particularly thick and homey. "Our brave troops," he would declare, "are on the march throughout the Middle East. The terrorists can run but they can't hide." A split screen would show Rangers rappelling out of Huey's on top of smoking mounds of earth. "We're gonna smoke 'em out of their holes," he would add. All the while, Bella would be churning away at the dirt, digging deeper for night crawlers.

At a critical point in the narrative, Dada would execute its typical volte-face of training the camera on the viewer. The poor bastard, wearing only boxers and a cut-off t-shirt, would be seated in his recliner, gazing dumbstruck at the TV while guzzling a beer. His right arm would be connected to an IV dripping mystery elixir into his veins. His eyes would be unblinking. The camera would focus on his hands. They would be swollen and inflamed and turning a bilious yellow. The skin rot was now on the move and nothing could stop it. It would soon be yellowing the carpet and fracturing the TV screen.

The camera would shift to Bella outside in the garden obsessively digging. Suddenly her ears would perk and she would freeze. Her gaze would be trained on something alarming in the dirt that she hadn't expected.

In early 2004, a White House spokesman defended the administration for providing the nation with moral clarity. In the same breath he noted that the Bush Administration "didn't do nuance" when it came to policy.

My first reaction was—that's interesting—no nuance. That would be like Ralph saying, "Let's just forget about the conflicting lab results and your confounding symptoms. Just for the hell of it, let's go directly to chemo."

I related my thoughts to Madeleine who was currently making a living as housecleaner. She immediately declared that she liked the concept. No more dirt for her either. The next day she was giving notice to her clients that she no longer dusted or vacuumed. It was simply too messy. Dirtless housecleaning—now there was a concept that any self-respecting Dadaist would have to appreciate.

In Dire Straits

Chapter 13

Bee Music

For nearly three years, a subtle drone-like music had been playing through most of my pain and discomfort, but I had been too preoccupied to notice. I suppose the first few notes were sounded in late 2001 by my naturopathic doctor in casually mentioning that several of his colleagues from John Bastyr Medical College were investigating the use of bee venom in treating arthritis. He offered me some literature and suggested that I might want to consider volunteering to be a guinea pig.

I gave it a quick scan and didn't find it very compelling. Mostly it consisted of anecdotal reports without supporting scientific evidence, which was never enough to pass my threshold of credibility. At the same time, the thought of bees swarming over my swollen joints wasn't exactly a comforting thought. It almost seemed medieval, which I suppose it was since it had been practiced for at least a millennium. Some reports dated it back to the time of Hippocrites. In any case, I decided just to stick with the antibiotics until I was sure one way or another whether they were working.

In Dire Straits

About a year later (in the fall of 2002) the next chord sounded when Madeleine dressed up Buffy in a bee suit for Halloween. This inspired much laughter and play, plus reminiscences that Gigi, Buffy's creator, took much delight in working in her garden in among joyfully buzzing bees and hummingbirds. An enduring memory was arriving at the old house in springtime and being greeted from afar with the words, "Come quick, an amazing hummingbird is at the feeder." It was always a great show. The visitors included the preciously tiny calliope male with red-ray throat markings, the male rufous with its handsome brown tail, and the regal Allen that could churn the wind into buttercream with its frenzied tail feathers.

Her delight in bees and hummingbirds came back to me anew when Madeleine suggested that I read Joel Rothschild's, *Signals*, a best seller that told the story of how he dealt with the loss of his partner and best friend Albert who died of AIDS. Apparently the two of them shared a great love of hummingbirds. A few days after finishing the book, I wrote Joel a letter, telling him about hummingbirds in my own past. I also shared a quote from Henry Miller's *Stand Still Like the Hummingbird*.

A week later Joel replied by e-mail, telling me just how much the quote meant to him. Apparently it expressed sentiments he shared with Albert and provided him with a lift during his current health crisis. Apparently he, too, was struggling with AIDS and might not survive it. To think that I could buoy someone else's spirit with a quote by Henry, whom I considered family, gave me a lift as well. I was glad that I had taken the time to write.

Henry Miller on Honey

When you find you can go neither backward nor forward, when you discover that you are no longer able to stand, sit or lie down, when your children have died of malnutrition and your aged parents have been sent to the poorhouse or the gas chamber, when you realize that you can neither write nor not write, when you are convinced that all exits are blocked, either you take to believing in miracles or you stand still like the hummingbird. The miracle is that the honey is always there, right under your nose, only you were too busy searching elsewhere to realize it. The worst is not death but being blind, blind to the fact that everything about life is in the nature of the miraculous.

Source: Henry Miller, *Stand Still Like the Hummingbird*

Winter of 2003 came and went with no more buzzing and wing beating by bees or hummingbirds, but then again I might have missed them because of my own focus on the war and my struggles with inflammation.

In spring of 2003, just after the operation, I decided to embellish the small shaded garden behind my apartment that for two years had been a meditative retreat. It already contained the grouted stone birdbath from my mom's garden. Enclosed by a high brick wall on one side and the face of my apartment building on the other, it received little direct sunlight and was always moist and cool. Because of this, it was dense with shade-loving plants including several species of fern, brilliantly yellow Irish poppies, delicate lavender campanula, and a profusion of leafy hosta, always the meal of choice for the local slug population.

The slugs were not alone in appreciating this cloistered

and dank Eden. Robins, chickadees, crows, thrushes, and sparrows regularly flocked to the birdbath and made their nests in the surrounding trees and dense camellia bushes. Figuring that one of them might enjoy an artful, handmade home, I installed one of my mom's birdhouses on the back wall and then a hummingbird feeder on an overhead support plank. Only a week later, I was surprised to discover that the birdhouse had been colonized by a swarm of honey bees—not exactly what I intended. In fact, I narrowly avoided a blinding sting when I peered inside the birdhouse.

The more I thought about this, the more I appreciated the serendipity of the buzzing homesteaders. Nature loved to overturn best-laid plans. It was only hubris to think that you could predict perfectly what would happen when you disrupted habitat. I just needed to be careful that I didn't stir up a storm.

Before revealing the next chord in the fugue, I should add that over the years I've paid increasing attention to coincidence. Travel has been the main persuader. On more than a few trips to Europe, I seemed to be guided by an invisible hand to just the right person, place, and opportunity. Of course, I hadn't traveled internationally for a long time, and maybe because of this was probably less attuned to coincidence.

This changed suddenly in fall 2004, when the universe essentially stung me out of my slumber. Just after Thanksgiving I made a resolution that despite my increasing inflammation and discomfort I would try to make more of an effort to connect with the outside world—at least get away to the local café and bookstore on occasion.

Although I had a couple of alternatives, my best option was Third Place Books and the adjoining Honey Bear Café. It was a convivial environment in which you were greeted at the door by an overlarge, cedar-wood bear holding a pot of honey. The café was at the back of the bookstore. The people who ran the combined establishment never pressured anyone to buy books or food and didn't even care if you borrowed a *New York Times*, *Nation* or *New Yorker* to browse over coffee.

On one of my first few visits, I reviewed the discouraging casualty news from Iraq and then turned my attention to the book review. One of the reviewers was gushing about a new novel by a promising young novelist. I was a little skeptical but decided it might be worth a look. A good novel was exactly what I needed to rekindle my own writing. After ten minutes I could only shake my head. There was nothing particularly insightful in the story. It was the epitome of minimalist fiction, focusing unreflectively on the struggles of samsara.

I tossed the book down and murmured, "I'll bet I can randomly discover something better." I closed my eyes, turned into a whirling dervish, and three revolutions later Buddha pointed my arthritic thirty-degree tilted finger at a book entitled, *The Secret Life of Bees* by Sue Monk Kidd.

I turned to the first page and read the following: "At night I would lie in bed and watch the show, how bees squeezed through the cracks of my bedroom wall and flew circles around the room, making that propeller sound, a high-pitched zzzzzzz that hummed along my skin. I watched their wings shining like bits of chrome in the dark and felt the longing build in my chest. The way those bees flew, not even looking for a flower, just flying for the feel of the wind, split my heart down its seam...Looking back on it now, I want to say the bees were sent to me. I want to say they showed up like the angel Gabriel appearing to the Virgin Mary, setting events in motion I could never have guessed."

I couldn't put it down and ended up reading most of it standing in place. It told a marvelous story of the relationship between a young white southern woman named Lily and three black beekeeping sisters who took her in. Essentially a story about orphanage and the healing power of love and forgiveness, the book seemed to derive much of its power from the connections to bees and beekeeping. Each chapter began with some interesting fact or observation about bees that related to events that followed.

On the Importance of the Queen Bee

A queenless colony is a pitiful and melancholy community; there may be mournful wail or lament from within...Without intervention, the colony will die. But introduce a new queen and the most extravagant change takes place.

Source: *The Queen Must Die: and Other Affairs of Bees and Men* (quoted from *The Secret Life of Bees* by Sue Monk Kidd)

The importance of the queen bee to the hive immediately triggered reflection about my mom's ever-ready support for anyone she felt needed some tender loving care. These included not only members of the extended family but neighbors, ex-wives trying to recover from a relationship, at least one unhappy adopted child, and more than a few artists beginning to doubt their own ability and vision.

Another theme in the story was about the importance to the spirit of purposeful work, which Lily gained in tending to the bees. Sue Kidd noted that bees without flowers grew listless and disoriented, but if the plants around them began to bloom they perked to life and showed boundless dedication. This reminded me of the fact that I always felt best about myself when I was hard at work creating something, be it art or books, or at least teaching. I wasn't doing any of this anymore. I had even shelved my anti-war efforts. I guess I was the listless, disoriented worker bee that Sue Kidd had described.

Bees and honey-making were much on my mind for the next twenty-four hours. Perhaps because of this, I decided to go back to my files and take a second look at the old information from my naturopath about bee-venom therapy. I had only been looking at it for a few minutes when I realized how much I had missed.

My oversight included several articles from a pain institute in New Jersey headed by Christopher M. Kim, M.D. One article summarized a study appearing in the French journal, *Rheumatologie* (March 1989), which reported a successful trial among 108 rheumatoid or osteoarthritis patients who hadn't responded to conventional treatments. Each patient was injected with bee venom by syringe, twice a week for six or more weeks, and all showed marked reduction in pain and swelling.

Other literature indicated that eighty to ninety percent of arthritis patients were significantly helped by the therapy and a high percentage experienced remission. Bee venom was apparently both a powerful anti-inflammatory and immune system modulator. Scientists had actually fractionated venom and found that it contained a number of enzymes and peptides beneficial to joints, the cardiovascular and immune systems. These included melittin, hyaluronidase, and cardiopep. Melittin stimulated the pituitary-adrenal axis and released both catecholamines and cortisol (the body's natural anti-inflammatory). Melittin also decreased arterial pressure and could be useful against arterial hypertension. Hyaluronidase was related to hyaluronic acid that lubricated joints. Cardiopep benefited the heart and also stimulated the adrenals.

Collective Mission of Bees

Honeybees depend not only on physical contact with the colony, but also require social companionship and support. Isolate a honeybee from her sisters and she will soon die.

Source: *The Queen Must Die: and Other Affairs of Bees and Men* (quoted from *The Secret Life of Bees* by Sue Monk Kidd)

Unfortunately, no one had yet found a way to separate the sting effect from the benefits of the venom. There were many unknowns, but the benefits of treatment were documented for over fifty disorders. These included a number of autoimmune and rheumatoid diseases.

After additional research, I learned that the therapy was most popular in Russia, Europe, India, and China, but had long been practiced in New England. Over two thousand articles had been written on the subject, mostly in Europe. Among the

American and Canadian M.D.s either endorsing or practicing the therapy were J. Broadman, Andrew Weil, Dietrich Klinghardt, Christopher M. Kim, Gerald Weissman, Joseph Saine, Glenn Rothfield, Rick Marinelli, and my own doctor, Ralph Golan.

The more I read, the more I was impressed. Bee venom had been found to be one hundred times more potent as an anti-inflammatory than hydrocortisone. Bee venom and its fractions also reduced pain by blocking the transmission of stimuli to peripheric and central synapses in the nervous system. The testimonials from M.D.s almost always reported a large majority of rheumatoid patients benefiting from the therapy. Severe allergic reactions, which people commonly worried about, only affected about two percent of the general population, but didn't present a significant problem in supervised therapy because doctors usually started slowly and mitigated anaphylactic shock with Benadryl and injectable adrenalin. In centuries of use, no fatalities had ever been recorded.

The side-effects of bee venom appeared to be minimal, mostly consisting of transient swelling, itching, and occasional dizziness. There were contraindications, however. Unrestricted use wasn't advised for pregnant women, patients with advanced cardiovascular complications, people with tuberculosis, various venereal diseases, diabetes, hepatitis, prostate enlargement, adrenal gland insufficiency, kidney insufficiency, and several other problems.

Within a few days, I visited Ralph Golan and we were soon on the phone conferencing with a Canadian expert on the therapy, a gruff and willful Russian émigré named Yevgheny who seemed like a character out of Gogol or Tolstoy. It quickly became apparent that he possessed an encyclopedic knowledge of therapy and every aspect of bees and honey.

Select Disorders Treated with Bee Venom

1. **Skin:** *acne, eczema, psoriasis, tropical ulcers, degranulating wounds, corns and warts, seborrheic dermatitis*
2. **Infections:** *laryngitis and mastitis. VIRAL: herpes simplex 1 and 2, post-herpetic neuralgia (shingles) and warts*
3. **Rheumatological:** *rheumatiod arthritis, osteoarthritis, juvenile rheumatoid arthritis, traumatic arthritis, ankylosing spondylitis, psoriatric arthritis, tennis elbow and bursitis rheumatic fever*
4. **Cardiovascular:** *hypertension (chronic and acute), arrhythmia, atherosclerosis, peripheral vascular disease, varicose veins*
5. **Pulmonary Disease:** *(COPD), bronchial asthma, emphysema*
6. **Sensory:** *hearing loss, vision, glaucoma, diplopia, iritis*
7. **Orthopedic:***slow bone healing, tendonitis, bursitis*
8. **Psychological:** *depression and mood swings*
9. **Endocrine:** *PMS, menstrual cramps, irregular periods, decreased blood sugar*

Source: American Apitherapy Association, Dr. Christopher M. Kim, M.D., *Managing Pain and Stress*, Fall 1986

"Of course, it will work for psoriatic arthritis," he declared when Ralph momentarily interrupted with the critical if somewhat impudent question. Our ears were soon buzzing with more information than we could possibly absorb, but we listened because we were supposed to, because this was what lowly peasants and doctors alike did when an authoritative Russian, wise in the ways of bees, explained their curative powers, which themselves could only be comprehended in the larger context of the Good Earth and Mother Russia. And there were profound lessons about spirit here as well that shouldn't be glossed over: bees were hardworking and fastidious, and so, too, was a good beekeeper, who always paid close attention to mood of his bees and the overall health of the hive. Were we paying attention?

He hoped we were, because we were talking about life force, and the need for austerity and discipline, which Tolstoy understood perhaps better than anyone.

"Tolstoy?" I murmured.

"Yes, it is imperative for the patient to practice rigor and austerity in diet, because the venom will not work to its full potential if you are dissolute and weak." He quickly rattled off a series of do's and don'ts that made more than a little sense.

Yevgheny ended the call abruptly. His bees were calling.

I turned to Ralph. "I think I'm going to like this therapy." Ralph grinned.

We passed the first test-injection without problem: no anaphylactic shock. I could almost hear Yevgheny declare, "This is good sign—patient not swell up like ripe tomato and die a miserable death. Very good. Nastrovia!"

I thought we might wait a few days for a regular set of injections, but Ralph was sure I would be OK, so we began injecting my larger joints. The pain was intense, but lasted only briefly followed by profuse sweating.

The next few sessions were increasingly difficult because we added more injections and began stinging my hands and feet, which were far more sensitive. When the pain was particularly intense, I gritted my teeth and muttered

"Nastrovia." At the end of a session I would sometimes shake like a leaf for thirty minutes and then quiver off and on for hours. Later in the evening a slight fever would set in, followed by a speeded-up brain that made me feel like a worker bee on steroids.

After a few more sessions, itching began and then worsened dramatically. If I could have, I would have shed my skin. I wanted to dull the sensation with aspirin or Benadryl, but the Russian advised against this, so I relied on cold baths and ice packs, except that they only helped for a few minutes and then the itching returned in force. Fortunately, the torture dropped off after the second day and usually this coincided with a dramatic reduction in my swelling. As the hours passed, I could actually see definition return to my fingers; I could see veins and folds of skin where before there was nothing but a puffy mass. The effect was more dramatic than anything I had experienced with prednisone or NSAIDs. Of course, this was about the time that I had to go in for another treatment. I was taking two to three a week and they were coming in such quick succession that it was hard to determine whether I was actually improving or simply riding a roller coaster of increasing and decreasing inflammation.

Nonetheless, the reduction in transient swelling fortified my resolve to continue. It helped also that Ralph was such a supportive doctor. He never flinched and was never hurried about forcing a needle on me despite the fact that I was taking up more of his time than I was paying for.

Sometimes black humor would keep us going. "Do it to me," I might say when I was ready for a painful injection in my hands, and he would grin like Dr. Zhivago's evil twin.

"Nastrovia." He would declare as the injection brought tears to my eyes.

"The Czar wears women's underwear," I muttered while wincing.

"Impudence. Next time we switch to wasp venom from Kharkov."

Charlyn, who had heard the ruckus from the front desk, arrived at the door to see what was going on. She spotted me sitting in a chair wearing only shorts. My back, feet hands and shoulders were dotted with traces of blood, and my eyes tearing. Ralph was poised over me with a raised syringe.

"Is everything OK?" she asked.

"We're going to need a fifth of Stoly here, Natasha."

"Da, ze dog will bring it," she deadpanned, closing the door behind her.

I suppose this silliness should come as no surprise. After all, these were people who had fed worms to their animals. Czarist swine. Come the Revolution, everything would change —patients would hold the syringe and doctors would be cowering before them in their underwear.

In Dire Straits

Chapter 14

Stings of Awareness

The therapy lasted ten weeks and took a heavy toll on my sleep and already limited energy. Madeleine gave me much encouragement, turning our play with Buffy and the bears in a new direction. When I was out getting stung, she would leave assignments on my answering machine. Everyone had a job to do. Buffy, as queen bee, should make sure that the worker bees assigned to sting me offered their most powerful venom; and the bears, at least for the moment, should curb their appetite for honey and make no raids on the hive.

Around the six-week mark, I noticed that the pain in my left shoulder was lessening and this was followed by reduced inflammation in joints that hadn't been "stung." At around the nine-week mark, at least ten of the injected joints were better, which left about twelve the same. This was improvement far beyond anything I had experienced in taking antibiotics. I might have been even more encouraged but for the fact that my morning dizziness and fatigue had worsened considerably.

Ralph thought I might have overloaded my adrenals, which Yevgheny had mentioned as a possible side effect of the venom. As Ralph explained it, "Just like a tired horse, exhausted adrenal glands will only grow weaker if they are continually overstimulated, overstressed, and whipped into action." The injections had offered the latest whipping and now I seemed to be caught up in a cycle of exhaustion and disrupted sleep that only further stressed my system.

To resuscitate the horse, Ralph prescribed a small amount of cortef (a supplement to natural cortisol) along with regular doses of vitamins B and C. These would compensate for the additional stress until my adrenals could catch up and recover.

Within a few weeks I was already feeling more energetic and clear-headed. This coincided with continued improvement in my joints. Apparently, the venom was still working its magic weeks after the last injections. I could now hold my neck up in the morning without pain killers, use my computer without straining my wrists, and perform such simple domestic chores as lifting groceries and washing dishes. I could even take short walks. I was sure that if I continued to improve, there was a good chance that I would be able to bicycle again, which would be a great tonic for my spirit.

I visited Ralph briefly and right away he could tell how much better I was moving and feeling. What neither of was certain of was whether to start a new round of injections and if so how long to wait. We decided to call Yevgheny.

He was full of the usual bravado when he answered the phone. No, he wasn't the least bit surprised by my progress. "Isn't this what I promised?"

"Well, yes," we both murmured deferentially in chorus.

176

"And you would advise a second round?" asked Ralph.

"Yes, of course, but only after a two-month recovery period."

"Well, this is terrific," answered Ralph.

"Yes, it is," replied Yevgheny with a tinge of mockery.

This became our plan along with a return to Dr. Brown's antibiotic regimen.

Six weeks after the injections ended, I noticed a slight regression in my condition. My hands and feet—the first joints to be struck by the disease—were somewhat inflamed, and a few of the larger joints had also grown sensitive.

I couldn't help but think of the Oliver Sacks's *Awakenings,* which told the story of Parkinson's patients benefiting from L-dopamine, but only temporarily. Eventually they lapsed back to stony rigidity. I didn't think a similar regression was likely, but was anxious to solidify my gains by starting the second round of injections.

Soon after they began, I received a phone call from my best friend in college, Steve Mikesell, who currently lived in California. Steve had grown up on a ranch in Boise and fit perfectly the image of the poet-cowboy—chiseled face, few words, quick wit. He would soon be in Seattle for a visit and hoped we could get together to catch up.

It had actually been some time since we had last seen each other. He knew nothing about my illness and I decided to tell him, even mentioning the bee venom.

He shot me a strange look.

"Damn," he replied. "I can't imagine dealing with something like this. Bee venom? Sounds god-awful."

I hemmed and hawed and said something to the effect that at first it was difficult but that I was getting used to it.

After Steve departed I realized that this wasn't exactly the truth.

You never really got used to the stings. I cringed with every injection and then waited for the onslaught of the pain, which always followed in about two seconds. Then I tried to breathe my way through it until it was time for the next joint injection.

I recalled what Sue Kidd had said about it: "Once you get stung, you can't get unstung." All you could really do was try to get over it and maybe learn something in the process.

One of the most poignant lessons imparted by disease is that you are more than the body ravaged and weakened by illness. As Gary Zukav describes it, the body is simply the house that the spirit lives in during its stay on the earth plane.

The notion of being more than your body was imparted during every set of injections. If the stings didn't immediately follow one another, I actually felt a strange disembodied sensation about thirty seconds later. It was narcotic-like and analgesic. A part of me seemed to be observing the affair with curious, almost disembodied amusement. I was reminded of Michael Murphy's accounts of Hindu ascetics who could withstand all manner of physical discomfort and deprivation by achieving a detached, above-the-fray witness state.

On the nights after each session, it was near impossible to sleep. I was too hot, too speedy, and itchy. I possessed just enough attention to page through my small library of books on yogi masters, usually with the bears looking over my shoulder.

I read accounts from the *Yoga Sutra*, listing dozens of *siddhis*, or powers of the most advanced adepts. Claims were made of yogis altering their shape, passing through walls, appearing in several different locations simultaneously, and materializing objects out of thin air. The more credible investigations by Michael Murphy documented fakirs who could go a month or more without food or water, and who could arrest their own heartbeat and vital signs and then switch them back on.

The bears weren't at all surprised by this, especially Fergie, my own honey bear who confided that he had been stung by bees his entire life and succeeded in achieving "witness" to reduce the pain. Other powers soon manifested, including an ability to materialize soluble fish.

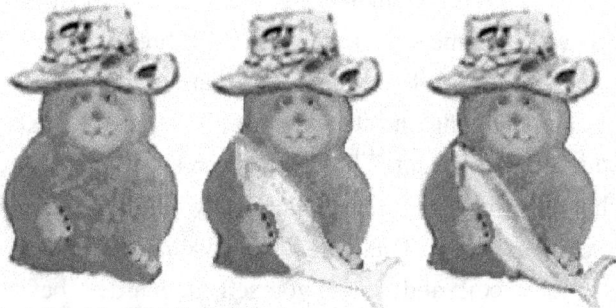

Fergie Materializes a Soluble Fish © Jim Currie

"Soluble fish?"

He only grinned knowingly.

I was skeptical, but I later saw him do this with my own eyes. Fortunately, a camera was handy and I was able to record the impressive demonstration. Quite clearly I had fallen in with a group of extraordinary bears, which I was sure improved my chances of benefiting from the bee venom.

Yes, I loved the entire concept of the therapy—not just the fact that it was cheap and unconventional, dating back a few thousand years, but that the sting was considered inseparable from the healing. Dr. Brown pointed this out in his book—the sting caused a fire alarm, ushering in the body's own fire fighters. They not only doused the joints that had been stung, but every other fire that might have been burning.

During the injections, when the pain began to spike, Ralph would advise me to breathe deeply, and this often softened the pain. I always wondered why this helped. It even helped on those nights after the injections when I didn't think I could endure the itching and fever.

Clearly oxygen intake made organs perform better, but I wondered if there might not be a spiritual element working here as well. I came across the notion that breath to the Greeks was *pneuma* or spirit. Dating back to antiquity, the Gnostics, yogis and Qigong masters have all believed that deep breathing could "inspire" healing and creativity. It dawned on me that the effects might be explained by letting go—the act of release in exhaling. Each breath was almost a test of your ability to uncoil and leave yourself unguarded before the forces of the universe.

"Nastrovia," was the toast that Ralph and I offered during the most difficult moments of bee venom therapy. But pain was never what we were really toasting. It was the chance to rise above the fear and suffering. As Larry Dossey stated, "Illness always asks a larger question: What is the mode of being in which I will take my stand during this illness—the local mode of isolated individual self or the nonlocal mode of the expanded, unitary Person, the state of One Mind, which is not limited to the here and now? In the end, sickness is always a question of being."

I only wished that the entire country had taken a few deeper breaths before rushing off to war. As a character in Michael Moore's film *Fahrenheit 911* declares, "You can make people do anything when they are afraid." He might have added—when they are contracted, rigid, and untrusting.

Not only will they do anything, they will see whatever they must to make themselves feel safer. In the process, they will turn the truth upside down and inside out, celebrate fools as heroes and vilify the people who carry candles into the darkness. Dada figured this out in the early 1900s, even before the world sent its sons off to the Flanders Field in another war that never should have been fought.

In Dire Straits

Chapter 15

Blues Brothers

Even though supplementation with cortef helped me recover from the injections, my adrenals and thyroid were still underperforming and this made me subject to mood swings. Grim news from the outside world exacerbated this, especially reports of increasing violence in Iraq, revelations of US torture and cover-up, and Bush Administration stonewalling on climate change. As one of my favorite political commentators put it: if you aren't upset or angry, you aren't paying attention.

In April 2004, photographs were revealed of Iraqi prisoners at Abu Ghraib Prison being tortured and humiliated by their American overseers. The Administration pinned responsibility on low-level soldiers and insisted that the Geneva Convention had not been violated or that higher-ups were involved. In the same month, Shiia uprisings led by the cleric Moqtada al-Sadr, began throughout Iraq. Soon these spread to Baghdad and Najaf.

Maybe because my energy and adrenals had been depleted by bee venom, I found it hard to be hopeful. It didn't help that John Kerry was running such a bad campaign against

George Bush, in particular, failing to confront the Swiftboaters. It didn't make any sense. His silence and detachment only gave credence to their claims and suggested that he could easily be bullied. I now began to dread the possibility that Bush and Cheney and their klatch of Constitution abusers, climate-change deniers, torture defenders, and character assassins would be reelected.

In November 2004, after election irregularities in Ohio that included widespread disenfranchisement of Black voters, George Bush was declared the winner by the networks. Aware of the evidence of what had occurred in Ohio, John Kerry made no protest and quickly conceded. I could only shake my head and try to calm the irate bears who were looking for someone to bite.

On January 2, 2005, just before the inauguration, a massive tsunami welled up from deep within the Indian Ocean and swallowed parts of Thailand, Java, Sri Lanka, and East Africa. For some reason, I took this particularly hard, especially the pictures of decimated villages and habitat. It was as if a nuclear bomb had struck. More than anything this seemed to punctuate the power of nature and the susceptibility of people and animals in harm's way.

The initial US pledge to help was feeble and half-hearted. It seemed almost crazy for political reasons alone, for this was a Muslim nation and offering help without any strings attached was exactly what you wanted to do to stem the rising world antipathy toward America, the country that had sanctioned torture against Muslims at Abu Ghraib and justified the attack on Iraq with fabricated claims of a WMD threat.

It wasn't lost on me that the areas hit hardest were coastal population centers. The sea had simply swallowed the land and made short shrift of any buildings. The devastation could be likened to extreme flooding and storms likely to become more prevalent with climate change.

On my better days when energy was high, I devoted more and more attention to the latest evidence on global warming, the work of IPCC (Intergovernmental Panel on Climate Change) and other research groups. Credible predictions suggested widespread extinctions caused by ocean acidification, changes in vegetation and land cover, glacier melt, sea-level rise, and extreme weather and drought. Low-lying areas were particularly at risk. In the US, these included Florida, New Orleans, parts of Mississippi, the Texas Gulf Coast, and estuaries of all the great rivers emptying into the ocean.

The Bush Administration had consistently refused to acknowledge the severity of the threat, human activities as a central driver, and the imperative to act quickly to lessen world-wide suffering and species loss. The Republican think tanks and supporters in the media were more vehement and routinely called predictions of climate change a hoax or a fraud. Despite my illness and limited attention span, it wasn't hard to see through the anti-intellectual polemic.

Back in 2003 James Hansen, head of the Goddard Institute for Space Studies, professor at Columbia University and one of the foremost climate experts, published a paper entitled, *Can We Defuse the Global Warming Time Bomb?* in which he noted, "Given the present unusual global warming rate on an already warm planet, we can anticipate that areas with summer melt and rain will expand over larger areas of Greenland and fringes of Antarctica. This will darken the ice surface in the season when the sun is high, promote freeze-thaw ice breakup, and, via ice crevasses, provide lubrication for ice sheet movement. Rising sea level itself tends to lift marine ice shelves that buttress land ice, unhinging them from anchor points. As ice shelves break up, this accelerates movement of land ice to the ocean."

In a 2004 presentation at the University of Iowa, he revealed that high-ranking officials in the Bush Administration were trying to stifle him from speaking out on anthropogenic "interference of the climate system."

The catastrophic images of glaciers melting, sea-level rising, pack ice declining, coral reefs acidifying, polar bears drowning, and elephants dying of associated drought were almost more than I could take. I wanted to do something about it—perhaps create an organization of old college classmates to publicize the threat, but I knew that my own healing crisis was still much in doubt. On further reflection, I decided that it would be a mistake to start something that exhausted me and maybe undermined my ability to live up to commitments. I needed to be soberly realistic and certainly not fight battles that I wasn't yet prepared for.

It was clear that with bee venom I had dampened my inflammation and maybe reduced the frequency of the storms. What was less clear was whether I was killing the bacteria I believed were the root cause of my problems. Despite some improvement, I still suffered from joint soreness, weakness, fatigue, digestive problems, sleep disorder, endocrine imbalance, and mood swings. A continuing problem that also frustrated me was that my hands were permanently damaged and limited my time at a keyboard.

Since my last round of bee venom, I had started taking antibiotics again. In my most objective assessment of Herxheimer versus disease pathology, I had to conclude that only a portion of my symptoms could be ascribed to the former. Dr. Trentham's words kept coming back to me that psoriatic arthritis didn't respond as well to antibiotic therapy as did rheumatoid.

A few months after George Bush's second inaugural, I decided to invest more energy in health research and after only a week discovered chatter on the internet about an interesting new approach to dealing with autoimmune diseases called the Marshall Protocol. Developed by Trevor Marshall, PhD, an Australian scientist recovering from sarcoidosis, it built on the basic theory of Dr. Brown, suggesting that l-class bacteria were the root cause of the diseases.

It went one large step further, asserting that bacteria infected immune-system cells (macrophages). It also made the distinction between inter and intra-cellular infection. The bacteria were so difficult to eradicate because they invaded and encysted themselves inside the nuclei of their hosts. Here they were both hard to detect and hard to destroy. The body's main response was to flail away at the invaders by releasing inflammatory cytokines that tended to isolate the infection, but in the process destroyed connective tissue. According to Marshall, a key factor in their persistence was that they interrupted the synthesis of antimicrobial peptides, which the body normally produced for protection and self-defense.

I could see that if all this were true, it explained many of the holes and ambiguities in Doctor Brown's discussion in the *Road Back*. He had offered no real answer as to why mycoplasma couldn't be rooted out by the immune system, how exactly the bacteria parasitized healthy cells, and how they were eradicated by antibiotics.

Marshall possessed an armamentarium of new investigative tools unavailable to Dr. Brown that supported his contentions. These included dark field microscopy to inspect the shape-shifting microbes, better understanding of cell receptors, and powerful new models in molecular biology that showed which chemicals, natural substances, and medicines up-regulated or down-regulated cell metabolism.

I found the research fascinating as well as difficult. I was even motivated to review old chemistry books so that I could better understand complex journal articles and nuanced drama of how microbes and immune cells tried to defeat each other. The remedy for this kind of infection, according to Dr. Marshall and agreeing with Dr. Brown, was to fortify the immune system, not disable it as mainstream rheumatology suggested. It was also necessary to disrupt the reproductive metabolism of the bacteria by interrupting protein synthesis and microbe replication.

Marshall called for the use of several antibiotics in a phased progression to amplify the body's assault on the elusive microbes. You started out with a single antibiotic to root out the least robust bacteria and moved on to the full cocktail in fighting the real Nazis. All the while you were taking an angiotensin receptor-blocker (Benicar) to disrupt genetic replication of bacteria and promote the work of antimicrobial peptides.

There was one other notable addition: Marshall called for the reduction of Vitamin D—more of a steroid than a vitamin—which molecular modeling had shown could inhibit the ability of antibiotics to kill cell-wall deficient bacteria. Keeping the Vitamin D down meant reducing exposure to sunlight and restricting foods such as fish and eggs.

I scheduled an appointment to talk with Ralph about this and presented him with the case. "Case" was the operative word because I brought along at least two pounds of journal articles, flyers, and results of the latest molecular modeling. I also came loaded with detailed histories of people benefiting in ways they never had from other protocols.

Ralph was impressed, but was quick to add that the detailed molecular biology was beyond his ken and something he didn't feel qualified to assess. The main issue, however, was risk. Both of us wanted to be sure that taking Benicar at an off-label dose didn't cause side-effects. Satisfied by the data, we decided to run a test of Vitamin D levels. Marshall had made the distinction between precursor form of Vitamin D (25-D) and its hydroxylated metabolite (1,25 D) that had been linked to immune system effects. He believed that a wide divergence between the two indicated a metabolic imbalance and likely intracellular infection, in which case you were a candidate for the protocol. We ran the test and the results suggested I fit the profile.

Following the Marshall Protocol required no small investment of energy and discipline—a far cry from taking antibiotics a few days a week as I had with Dr. Brown's protocol. First, I had to reduce the sunlight in my apartment by covering the windows. In effect, I was turning my own quarters into a cave, which much amused the bears and the Buddha. The Buddha, in fact, briefly wondered whether I had abandoned the Middle Way and had thrown my lot in with the self-abnegating Hindu fakirs. I suppose I added to that suggestion when I took to wearing black pants and shirt, accessorized with wrap-around Noir sunglasses, and eliminated foods that contained Vitamin D, most notably fish, which briefly caused a riot among all the bears.

One of the main reasons I was drawn to the protocol was that many people reported that they were now for the first time experiencing an unmistakable herx. These included people afflicted with Lyme disease, Lupus, rheumatoid and psoriatic arthritis, Sjogren's, chronic fatigue, and fibromyalgia. At least three people were suffering from psoriatic arthritis. One claimed to be in total remission.

I had no idea just how profound the herx would be. As soon as I amped up to taking both Benicar and minocycline together, I was nearly leveled: my knees inflamed to the point I couldn't walk; muscle spasms erupted across my back; and my eyes were so sore I couldn't read, watch any television, or stare at a computer screen. But to my amazement, most of this abated within a few days. It was clear that this was a regimen you didn't rush: baby steps first.

Humor helped get me get through it. I cut the image of a

Blues Brother with my Noir glasses, long-sleeve black shirt, and Henry Miller fedora. Friends either thought I had slipped into abject fantasy or had turned anarchist in reaction to the election. Madeleine, Big Sydney, Buffy, and the Buddha immediately read the potential for theater and changed their own wardrobes and accessories. Everyone wore dark glasses.

"We're all Blues Brothers now," declared the Buddha-hipster.

Madeleine was at first skeptical about the protocol but like me was impressed by the science. She too found the stories compelling of people getting better who never before had responded well to any kind of therapy.

So many of these people were very bright and seemed to possess a pioneer mentality. The community included engineers, doctors, nurses, and scientists—all of them ready to share their opinions, latest research and even help Dr. Marshall in the science. On a daily basis someone on the MP would be posting the latest photographic evidence of pleomorphic bacteria escaping a cell nucleus or a critical review of someone's study on cell receptors. If you needed help, you got it immediately.

Though there were basic guidelines available to patients and doctors, the protocol required a great deal of personal evaluation and adjustment. It was up to you to process your own response and decide whether to drop back to an earlier stage, stay the course, or advance. All of this fit my basic philosophy and that of Madeleine, as well, of being your own healer/co-healer and making a commitment to understand both the disease and healing process.

In Dire Straits

Madeleine capsulated it perfectly by offering a quote by George Sheehan, M.D. out of *This Running Life*: "I have two choices (with illness): to delegate authority for its management or to accept it myself. I can watch the doctor or assume command; see the doctor as the all-knowing doer or as a teacher and companion in this cooperative effort...The written word must be suspect...If you are going to rely on an expert, let him speak directly to you, and not through someone else. If you read about something outside your experience, be sure you read the original and not the commentary."

A good number of people joined the protocol and dropped out within the first year—at least twenty percent. This was understandable. It was very difficult and sometimes a little scary to cope with the symptoms and herx, particularly new symptoms such as neuropathy.

For the first time, I began experiencing myoclonic jerks (muscle twitching) and parasthesia (something akin to tingling in extremities). I might have been more alarmed but for the fact that others had reported something similar and said that they usually went away as you progressed. Ralph wasn't so sure and decided to review both listed side effects and contraindications. He came up empty: there just wasn't anything there.

I passed on some general remarks from Dr. Marshall that new symptoms often indicated that the protocol was working and that you were uncovering previously untouched bacteria. With some mutual reservations, we decided to proceed but with even closer monitoring: if possible I would try to determine if the neuropathy correlated with the timing or dosage of Benicar and antibiotics and whether it rose or fell in concert with other symptoms.

A main consideration for me was that I was willing to get worse in order to get better. That's what Dr. Brown had convinced me was necessary: l-class bacteria just didn't give up the ghost that easily. I knew also that when they died, they managed to spread the misery by flooding your system with toxins, suggesting, as a result, that you were actually getting worse from your disease.

It was a very sophisticated and clever evolutionary strategy that actually preyed on fear and alarm, just the sort I was sure Karl Rove and other propagandists within the Bush Administration would have appreciated. The worst thing you could do, however, was focus on the symptoms and try to dampen them with powerful immune suppressants and steroidal anti-inflammatories.

The challenge was to maintain your wits and stay mindful of the difference between disease and die-off. They were difficult but not impossible to disentangle. The related challenge that I was constantly mindful of was just how much worse I was willing to get before retreat to other remedies.

I did have a few options that included concoctions to clear toxins from blood and lymph systems and, of course, I could also call in the bears to release the bees. The bears were always in favor of that because they were sure that a bee that was stinging me was a bee that wasn't protecting the hive from honey-raiders.

After a couple of months, I began to grow more confident that the neuropathy wasn't worsening. In fact, I now began to think of it more as a nuisance and irritant than something to really worry about. Most of the myoclonic jerking seemed to occur when I was just about to fall asleep. Suddenly a leg or arm would twitch or, worst case, I would nail one of the bears dozing next to me. Fergie, Big Sydney, and the other bears got used to this. It didn't surprise me. After all, these were bears who had given up salmon, crab, and fresh trout on my behalf. The one thing I knew with certainty was that if all this sacrifice eventually paid off, I owed them big-time.

A main unresolved conflict with Marshall and my doctors involved endocrines. Marshall was convinced that hypothyroidism and adrenal insufficiency, two problems I was constantly fighting with, would self-correct as I improved. He frowned on taking steroids, including cortef, that might support the proliferation of bacteria. For Ralph and I, the issue wasn't whether endocrines would correct on their own, but what happened until they did.

Was I willing to risk these consequences? Effects of insufficiency, according to Ralph, included sleep loss, slow recovery from strained muscles and tendons, slow wound-healing, extreme fatigue, and lowered immune defenses. In Ralph's view, a distinction should be made between supplementing beyond normal levels and simply making up for a confirmed insufficiency.

I weighed the pros and cons and decided that I would test for deficits and then supplement as Ralph recommended. The guiding principle here would be: no more than necessary. I tried to be disciplined in my monitoring, keeping careful records of what I was taking, how much I was sleeping, and all the neuropathy, dizziness, and inflammation I was experiencing. I wasn't simply trying to document daily changes but establish trends. Ultimately it was the trend that mattered. It was much like the difference between climate change and weather. My intent was to establish the trends in climate, and not be distracted by storms or brief periods of equable calm.

On the climate front, shoulders, knees, and elbows didn't seem as sore as before, and I was gradually developing more strength and resilience. Only a year earlier, a stretch and yawn in the morning might have strained or torn a muscle or tendon. Back then I was like an over-strung banjo.

I did experience two significant monsoons. The first involved a suddenly swollen jaw that made it hard to eat. The inflammation wouldn't go away with the usual palliatives, so I decided to see a dentist. He poked and prodded and even took X-rays but could find no abscess. He was at a complete loss. I subsequently saw Ralph and he prescribed a strong detoxifying concoction containing chlorella. Within a week my symptoms abated and this only added to my conviction that I was killing bacteria and the symptoms I was experiencing were herx.

Then suddenly in late 2005, I developed kidney stones that didn't pass and had to undergo an operation to remove them. Even the professionals at the Marshall Protocol and Dr. Marshall himself seemed concerned about this. Ralph was especially apprehensive. Whether the stones were caused by the protocol, disease progression, or maybe even some unconsidered herx was uncertain—there was just no guidance here; no relevant patient histories. It seemed that once again I was back in the "cloud of unknowing." Rather than retreat I made the willful decision to plow ahead.

The bears offered support but didn't really seem to mind being in the cloud unknowing. On nights when I would thrash about restively, Fergie, Little Sydney, Big Sydney, and their friends would take to the sky in an airship of their own design and marvel at the clouds, floating noiselessly above mountains, valleys, and oceans.

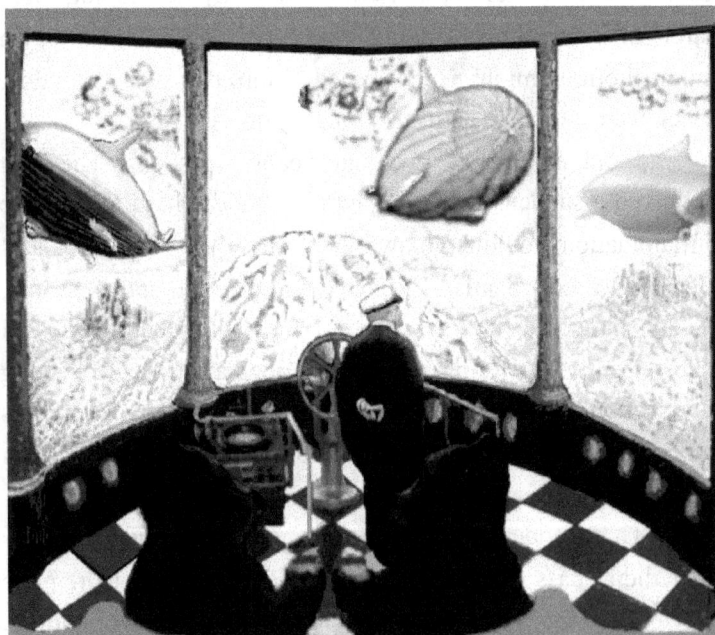

Inaugural Flight of Bearship 1.2 © Jim Currie

In the months that followed, I experienced no more stones and no more eruptions of jaw soreness. There were other smaller setbacks mostly involving joint inflammation, but I could tell that week-by-week I was getting stronger. My early-morning dizziness and irritability—perhaps my most intractable symptoms—had also improved slightly. I was now beginning to glimpse the possibility of life largely free from this debilitating disease.

In Dire Straits

Chapter 16

Listening to Elephants

By 2007, it was clear that my improvement was no short-term blip. Most of what Marshall predicted had come to pass. I was still experiencing hand problems, transient inflammation, morning dizziness, and strange neurological symptoms, but all seemed to fit the Marshall theory of bacterial die-off.

Month to month, most of my joints continued to improve. Shoulders, knees, and even wrists were only occasionally sore. Hands and feet remained a problem, and my lungs, oddly enough, would occasionally clog as they had just before I got sick in 2000. It was as if I was reversing the entire disease progression back to the onset of my grief and the attack by the stealthy microbe-terrorists.

I was now energetic enough to create a website called Sydney's Thumb (http://www.SydneysThumb.com) devoted to mindful travel and conservation. A main theme was to promote well body and well earth and show the links between them. I also wanted to show how the principles of cohealing could be practiced in protecting animals and ecosystems.

In Dire Straits

Back in the 1980s, The Sierra Club had produced a great book on the subject, showing the many ways in which the earth operated like the human body. Like the body, the biosphere depended on an extensive network of metabolic pathways, feedback mechanisms, systems for processing waste, and smart information processors. If you overloaded capacity (e.g., from a massive oil spill), you could expect disastrous consequences, including effects on species that weren't easy to reverse.

Most biologists believed that human beings were causing the greatest mass extinction of species since the dinosaurs vanished sixty-five million years ago. Now over one-fourth of all mammals were considered in trouble. If present trends continued, up to one-fifth of all species could disappear within thirty years and one half in one hundred years. This was the epitome of a healing crisis.

It even possessed a spiritual element as the noted biologist, E.O. Wilson, had pointed out. In fact, protection of the earth and animal kingdom was called for by most of the world's religions, with numerous mentions in the Holy books of Judaism, Christianity, Islam, Buddhism, Jainism, Hinduism, and Confucianism.

I was especially concerned about the "tipping-point problem," which I had witnessed in my own private realm when my combined stresses (in the year after my mom's death) were more than I could handle. This was a concept that related directly to CO_2 and global climate change.

James Hansen and his peers were ringing the alarm on this but American politicians, in particular, didn't seem to be listening. In Hansen's view we had already reached a tipping point (at around at 385 ppm CO_2) because of the melting of the Greenland and West Antarctica ice sheets and the recession of the Arctic ice cap. Each added positive, amplifying feedback to climate change.

His argument, supported by detailed quantitative analysis, was published in a 2008 journal article. He subsequently offered a summary in testimony before Congress: "The shocking conclusion...is that the safe sea level atmosphere carbon dioxide is no more than 350 ppm (parts per million), and it may be less. Carbon dioxide is already 385 ppm and rising about 2 ppm per year. Shocking corollary: the off-stated goal to keep global warming less than two degrees Celsius (3.6 degrees Fahrenheit) is a recipe for global disaster, not salvation."

The issue was overload and dramatic state-change, something I had experienced first-hand in my own health crisis. I was pretty sure that others could relate to this as well if the issue were presented in the right terms. Most everyone I knew understood that with inattention to toxic exposure, bad diet, and other stressors, you were living on borrowed time. Eventually, niggling sub-acute problems would go ballistic and then you were caught up in a runaway cycle that was hard to reverse—maybe even impossible.

I kept thinking about the impact on me of reading Ralph's book for the first time—discovering all the reinforcing and connecting pathways that related to inflammation and immune response. It seemed that James Hansen was really working to illuminate the same basic problem (i.e., homeostatic overload, inflammation and state-change) but just at a higher level of organization and integration.

What I appreciated most about his work was that besides the disciplined science, he "popped" the important questions about impediments to change and consequences. Few other scientists, or for that matter politicians, were willing to talk about this: what policy decisions and power relationships created this mess? Where should we place the burden of proof in assessing causality and future trajectories? What are the social costs, indirect and direct of the palliative solutions? What are the implications to quality of life under a dramatically altered climate regime? How will we explain our failure to act to future generations? How can we justify the mass extinctions that are sure to follow?

He was even making some of the same arguments for self-empowerment that George Sheehan, Larry Dossey, and Ralph Golan had made in discussing co-healing. In his testimony before Congress he stated, "If politicians remain at loggerheads, citizens must lead. We must demand a moratorium on new coal-fired plants. We must block fossil fuel interests who aim to squeeze every last drop of oil from public lands, off-shore, and wilderness areas. Those last drops are no solution. They provide continued exorbitant profits for a short-sighted self-serving industry, but no alleviation of our addiction or long-term solution." With a dose of imagination and substitution of phrasing, this could have been Thomas Brown appearing on the *Today Show* and addressing the blockade by the American Rheumatism Association and their defense of steroids and toxic drugs.

I appreciated the fact that good science alone wasn't going to mobilize the body politic to act on climate change. Politicians would have their say and mostly they followed rather than led. They were also at least as corruptible as the doctors who took the handouts and bribes of the pharmaceutical companies. The one thing that they cared about, however, was reelection and one thing they worried about was that their constituents would view them as out of touch and on the wrong side of important issues.

Therefore the audience of Sydney's Thumb had to be the public with the goal of mobilizing grass roots activism and pressure. The message also had to be as playful as it was scientific and analytical. Play and laughter was one of the great antidotes to fear, which defenders of the status quo were relying on to stymie opposition and public rage.

It wasn't lost on me that I never would have gotten this far in my own self-healing if I hadn't frequently relied on play to break the juggernaut of my worry about disability and inflammation. How many nights had I watched reruns of *Seinfeld* and laughed so hard that all anxieties fled?

If not for the charades and dramas with Madeleine, Buffy, and the bears, I'm sure I would have succumbed to the most paralyzing depression. My entire healing odyssey from the encounter with the cowgirl angel to Bella's scramble through the dirt and Yevgheny's bees was a testament to the power of exploration and unlikely association, mostly triggered by playfulness and laughter.

In the first week after Sydney's Thumb was launched, a coup occurred: the bears took over the website. Little Sydney became the subject of the logo, sitting on the top of a spinning globe and proudly holding his oversized hitchhiker's thumb high in the air.

This was our collective tribute to the evolutionary biologist, Stephen Gould, revered by all the bears for his famous book, *The Panda's Thumb*. The anti-intellectual proponents of intelligent design had corrupted the whole story behind the evolution of the panda's thumb, and it was important, just in honor of the now deceased Stephen Gould, to take it back.

A few days later, Fergie made a statement of his own, declaring that he wanted to open a virtual travel café for bears and mindful travelers. Since he was our largest and most easily agitated bear, no one disagreed and he was immediately appointed head "bear-tender" and chief carpenter.

Within a few days, he constructed a rotating neon-fish sign on the façade and began seating a motley group of fugitive bears, eccentric travelers, and loosely-wound artists at the bar. All patrons were subjected to his whoppers about the monster Chinook salmon that got away. All unapologetic supporters of the Bush Administration were immediately bounced from the premises.

A few weeks after the grand opening, we opened up new wings of the restaurant in the basement aquarium and then a jungle patio. The expansion might have been a little premature because a basking shark subsequently broke through the aquarium Plexiglas, causing bears and dining travelers to swim for their lives.

In the spirit of *The Mindful Traveler*, I challenged myself to create most of the artwork for Sydney's Thumb and to write the computer code. This was a major challenge given my lack of dexterity and physical limitations, but I was in no great hurry, and if soreness set in, I would just stand down. One step at time—just like Satish's mindful unhurried walk through the Kyber Pass and the Hindu Kush.

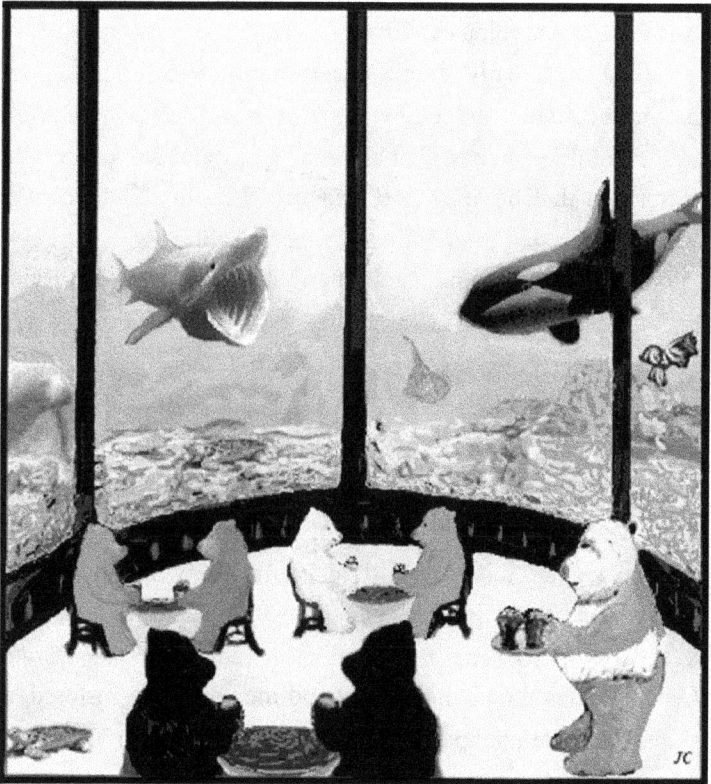

Calm Before the Storm in the Aquarium © Jim Currie

As the site began to take shape, I came across the inspiring words of one of my heroes, the unsinkable Howard

In Dire Straits

Zinn: "To be hopeful in bad times is not just foolishly romantic. It is based on a fact that human history is a history not only of cruelty but also of compassion, sacrifice, courage, kindness. And if we do act in however small a way, we don't have to wait for some grand utopian future. The future is an infinite succession of presents, and to live now as we think human beings should live in defiance of all that is bad around us is itself a marvelous victory."

The one really impressive virtue of Howard Zinn was that he refused to undone by anxieties that what he was doing might be futile. He just kept chipping away and working on the campaigns that he knew were needed. It didn't even seem to matter to him that often only a few people followed.

Now I think I understood why. The change he was trying to manifest wasn't just external. He was constructing his own reality and creating his own field. This, I was sure, was what he was talking it about when he spoke of the "infinite succession of presents." To embrace the present moment and still the noisy chatter were always the imperative when you were dealing with dire straits of any type. Once the deep listening began, it was usually just a matter of time before the thunderbolts of imagination began to strike begin to strike.

This made me think of the credo of *The Mindful Traveler*: to embrace the present and the challenges offered, to prepare for the unexpected and adjust accordingly. There was always some latent opportunity about to erupt if you were agile enough to pick up on it.

Among the stories in the first six months that affected us most deeply was the plight of elephants throughout the globe.

As reported by Gay Bradshaw, Charles Siebert, Cynthia Moss, and others, wild elephant populations worldwide were under serious stress. The combined effects of poaching, agricultural expansion into traditional elephant habitat, culling by wildlife agencies, capture by circuses, drought, and climate change, were not only decimating populations but intensifying elephant aggression which they were directing at both humans and rhinos they shared habitat with.

Gay Bradshaw, a psychologist at Oregon State University, made the case that we were witnessing a breakdown of elephant society. At first I was a little skeptical of projecting human social qualities and sensitivities upon elephants, but she won me over. She showed how elephants grieve, express gratitude and joy, occasionally suffer from depression, and might grow distraught, confused or enraged over the loss of a beloved infant, parent, or leader.

Adolescent male elephants seemed to be especially dependent on the guidance and wisdom of elders in learning how to control their aggression, but unfortunately fewer and fewer of the elders were surviving because of poaching. Clearly elephants were far more intelligent, emotional, aware, and vulnerable than I ever imagined.

The way they responded to grief probably affected me most. I learned that after a family member or baby died, the mother and other female elephants would often cover the body with earth or brush. The "elies" even conducted vigils next to a fallen loved one, rumbling an eerie, mourning evensong.

I soon found a video that brought an upwelling of tears. I watched the return of a female herd to the site where their much beloved matriarch had fallen years earlier. They hadn't forgotten her and in turn the elephants approached and gently nuzzled her bones.

A story from Thailand about a baby elephant named Boon Lott touched me like no other. Born several months premature, Boon Lott ("survivor" in Thai) had been transported with his mother, Pang Tong, to an elephant hospital in northern Thailand where a young volunteer named Katherine Connor took him under her wing. His precarious start in life had left him with a calcium deficiency and weak bones.

When Boon was six-months old, his owner decided to sell him to a tourist facility and put his mother back to work in the logging industry. Katherine knew Boon was too weak and dependent on his mother for that: he would never survive the separation. She immediately launched a fundraising campaign, "Save Baby Babar" to produce money to pay off the owner. Just enough money was raised to forestall the sale until Boon could be weaned and would have a fighting chance to survive.

Unfortunately, the baby elephant soon suffered a fall that left him paralyzed and unable to stand. Experts predicted he would die within a few days. Katherine wouldn't give up and was determined to help him recover. With her own funds exhausted, she again appealed to others for help and raised money for a hydrotherapy pool to improve his circulation. Then, after an exhaustive internet search, she learned of a device called an Anderson Sling used for horses that might support him while his legs healed. She sent for one and when it arrived, worked with a team to modify it for the baby elephant.

It seemed to work. Now the challenge was to increase Boon's strength and improve his circulation. Katherine set to work, giving him daily therapy of acupuncture and massage. The next major step was to help him walk but without putting too much pressure on his weak legs. Engineers from Chiang Mai University offered help, designing and fabricating the world's first elephant wheelchair.

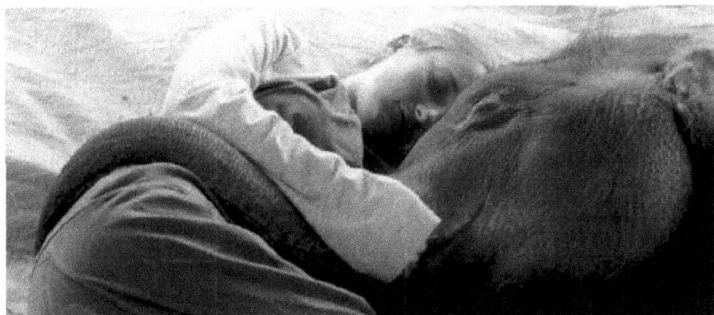

Katherine Connor at Side of Boon Lott © Katherine Connor

Katherine was elated to discover that it worked. Each day with Katherine hovering over him and offering encouragement, the indomitable baby elephant would struggle to his stand on his own and take a few bold-hearted steps.

Just when it seemed that he might fully recover, he fell again, this time snapping his femur in half. From this there would be no recovery even for such a willful and brave spirit. On June 26, 2004, with Katherine holding him close, Boon's valiant heart stopped beating. In honor of his great courage, Katherine established BLES (The Boon Lott Elephant Sanctuary) that is dedicated to elephant rescue and the world-wide protection of elephants. (http://www.blesele.org).

In Dire Straits

A few months after I came across the story, I contacted Katherine in Thailand and made a pledge that Sydney's Thumb would help the sanctuary in whatever way we could, if only to pass on word about all the good work she was doing. We would also make a significant commitment to the cause of elephant conservation and rescue, and the imperative to stop poaching and halt the circus abuse of elephants.

Despite the stories of tragedy and setback, Sydney's Thumb, with the bears in command, steered a positive and empowering course, relating stories of success as often as setback. We reported on orangutan rescue work in Borneo, panda conservation in Sichuan China, and the great veterinary work in Uganda by Dr. Gladys Kalema-Zikusoka in promoting One Health (the link between human and animal health).

The idea that imagination begets more imagination and creative problem-solving has been a guiding principle behind Sydney's Thumb. This has included artistic imagination to reflect and capture the unique spirit of place. Friends frequently forward stunning photography and dazzling paintings of wild places.

Most recently the bears made the suggestion that we publicize the importance of Pacific Northwest rain forests to planetary health and we faithfully rendered a secret place in the Olympic rainforest known to Sydney, Fergie, and the other bears as Bear Meadow. It has since become a virtual retreat for all Friends of Sydney's Thumb and a place to renew energy and resolve in promoting climate action, animal protection and a healthy and resilient biosphere.

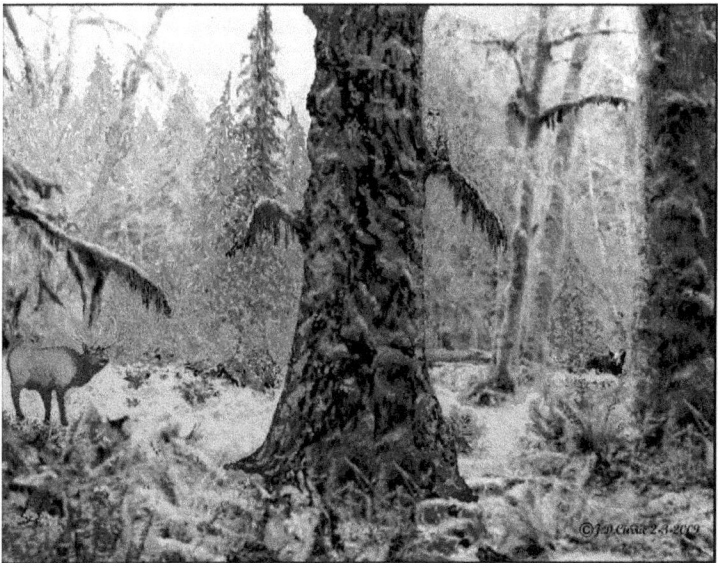

Bear Meadow © Jim Currie

In Dire Straits

Chapter 17

Spirit of the Fallen Matriarch

I had only visited Gigi's grave a few times since the funeral. Whenever I did, I fell into a deluge of grief that might last a day or more. I still communed with her spirit, however, and most often that took place in the sheltered garden behind my apartment, which I had turned into a postage-stamp wildlife refuge. It included her old grouted birdbath, as well as a wooden, handmade birdhouse that had been taken over by the bees.

Nearly every day I found at least a few minutes to sit or stand quietly at the base of the birdbath and watch honey bees tend tirelessly to the pollen-heavy campanula and the Irish papaver. When they could carry no more riches, they streaked for the birdhouse, which was always droning with activity.

Not far away was the hummingbird feeder. I had never actually seen a bird at the spout, but every few weeks I had to add nectar, so I was sure that honey-diviners were about, attracted by the handsome ruby-throat that my mom had painted on the glass.

Well into phase two of the Marshall Protocol, I

awakened one morning, checked the nectar, and then headed off to The Honey Bear Café where I planned to work on conservation issues. On my way out, I reached for Buffy who was overdue for a stay with Madeleine. I would drop her off on my way back home. She enjoyed The Honey Bear as well, particularly the attention she got from the female staff whenever I seated her next to me while reading the paper.

It was a brilliantly sunny, June morning, never to be taken for granted in Seattle, which probably explained why the café was empty except for a few employees. Most people weren't foolish enough to spend their time indoors unless a job required it or they were working on something inspired. I read the paper quickly, scanned the table of new releases at the front of the bookstore, and made my way to the car with Buffy. Stopping at a traffic light a few blocks later, I noticed a nearby yard verdant with new foliage. Several rose bushes were bowed from the weight of new blossoms and had strewn their petals tearfully across a thick carpet of unmowed grass. The recent rains must have created this surge of new growth. I only hoped that Gigi's grave marker wasn't completely covered. I had no idea how carefully the attendants watched over it.

Absorbed in thought about the condition of the grave, I missed my turn south toward Eastlake. A few blocks later, I realized I might as well visit the cemetery. It was only a few miles away. As I drew near the entrance, I felt an upwelling of the pandemonium from that dark winter day in late 1998, but it passed quickly, perhaps because it was so beautiful out. The aroma of cut grass was in the air and also the scent of lilac blossoms.

A few minutes later I was at graveside beneath a flowering elm tree. The marker was well defined. The caretakers had been fastidious in keeping the grasses at bay.

"Beloved wife, mother, enduring spirit," read the inscription on the simple marker. A freshet of tears welled up from my heart, and then another a few minutes later. With each passing minute I felt calmer and stronger. Bye and bye, I even began to feel light-hearted.

I was so glad that the cemetery was natural—a peaceful resting-place with many mature trees, and best of all, no gaudy tombs and vain vertical tombstones proclaiming how much people were loved and how much they had accomplished. The birds seemed to appreciate the habitat as well. I watched several squawking chickadees streak for the elm tree and then vacate it for a stately Douglas fir. A thrush sang out vaingloriously somewhere in its upper boughs, and I headed off to see if I could catch sight of it, leaving Buffy to chat with Gigi.

The dense canopy kept it hidden no matter where I stood, so I gave up and began passing along a row of markers, inspecting the inscriptions. At least half seemed to be scripted by the religious wing of Hallmark, mentioning the loving hands of Jesus or God's grace, but I was actually surprised by how many were personal and gave a hint of what a person's life was really about. After thirty markers, I discovered a woman dedicated to charity, then a minister committed to civil rights, and finally a beloved healer.

Just when I was sure that I had exhausted the most personal statements of meaning and spirit, I came to a new gravesite. Across the granite stone lay a single crimson rose covering the following words: "When the light within us reaches the sky." No clue was offered of the fellow's life work; no mention made of family, just the lyrical phrase on an unusual stone. The image reminded me of the last words ascribed to Goethe: "More Light." I took a deep breath of the lilac-scented air and felt a surge of energy pass from my heart outward to my hands, then another radiate to my gnarled toes.

I could see Buffy in the distance joyfully bending Gigi's ear, relating all the events that had transpired since they had last been together. I was hesitant to interrupt but knew that the time was ripe to get something done. No telling how long it would last. Gigi was probably anxious as well to begin mixing paints and work on her latest landscape. There always seemed to be a canvas on her easel, if only an old painting she hoped to bring to life with a different pitch from the overhead sun. Perhaps today on Sydney's Thumb I would write about hummingbirds, the nature paintings of Sky Carpenter, and the secrets of Luminists floating high above in the radiant ether.

Epilogue

In 2009 and 2010, Sydney's Thumb continued to report on important environmental issues with a special focus on climate change, biodiversity, ocean impacts, and elephant protection. My improving health made it possible to devote more attention to this though I did experience occasional setbacks that made me realize that I wasn't completely out of the woods.

The bears at Sydney's Thumb didn't think that this was necessarily a bad thing and continued to make journeys of their own to Bear Meadow and the skies above Mount Rainer in Bearship 1.2. In sleepy-time hours they prodded me with visions that took form in new website artwork.

On April 22, 2010, the gross negligence of British Petroleum combined with inadequate government and Congressional oversight resulted in the Deepwater Horizon Oil Gusher that threatened to turn the Gulf of Mexico into a toxic soup, destroy nursery wetlands, and extinquish species that were already suffering the effects of climate change, uncontrolled land use, water pollution, coral reef loss, and ocean acidification.

The despair at Sydney's Thumb was nearly paralyzing. In a moment of consternation we returned to the words of Howard Zinn and realized that we had to respond in some fashion, no matter how small and seemingly inconsequential.

On June 14, we happened to view a CBS News story by Steve Hartman telling of an eleven-year-old girl so distraught over the death of Gulf turtles and pelicans that she decided to create artwork and sell it to help save animals. Light bulbs flashed and the bears began jumping and waving their arms: couldn't Sydney's Thumb add to this great idea?

The next day we began contacting prominent artists, musicians, writers, and film-makers to see if they, too, would be willing to participate and sell their works to support animal rescue.

All the immediate responses were positive. Within days a new effort was launched by Sydney's Thumb: *Artists for Oceans and Animal (AOA)*. It would be a vanguard effort by artists to support animal rescue and to protect oceans, wildlands, and endangered species. The crisis in the Gulf would be the initial focus.

Artists would give a percentage of proceeds from the sales of their work to support the people on the front lines who were rescuing and nursing oiled pelicans, cranes, dolphins, and other affected species. Money would also go to the groups that I was already working with to protect the Arctic, coral reefs, and other critical habitats from oil and gas exploration, misguided land use, shipping, and greenhouse gases.

At the heart of this commitment lay the realization

among artists that wildlands from the Okavengo to Prince William Sound are indispensable to their own artistic inspiration. They could demonstrate this with tangible contributions. Their patrons and supporters could do the same by purchasing designated AOA works (typically graced by the AOA Pelican). This wasn't simply about raising money and placing it in the right hands. It was about electrifying collective response to arrest climate change, putting pressure on people in power, and ushering in new and more mindful leaders who didn't simply mouth their concern for the commons.

I wasn't sure where AOA might lead, but I knew with perfect certainty that it was a necessary step to potentiate the field. No doubt there would be a succession of unexpected presents that would lead to even more fertile and conductive terrain. This seemed to be the kind of contribution that Howard Zinn would have endorsed and it was a perfect tribute to my own mom's great love of hummingbirds, oceans, and wildlands.

In Dire Straits

Recommended Readings

Bensen, Herbert. *Timeless Healing*. New York: Scribner, 1996.

Berman, Morris. *Coming to Our Senses*. New York: Bantam, 1990.

Berman, Morris. *The Twilight of American Culture*. New York: W.W. Norton and Company, 2000.

Chopra, Deepak. *Quantum Healing*. New York: Bantam, 1990.

Chodron, Pema. *The Places That Scare You*. Boston: Shambhala, 2001.

Chodron, Pema. *When Things Fall Apart: Heart Advice for Difficult Times*. Boston: Shambhala, 2000.

Currie, Jim. *The Mindful Traveler: A Guide to Journaling and Transformative Travel*. Chicago: Open Court, 2000.

Dass, Ram and Gorman, Paul. *How Can I Help?* New York: Alfred Knopf and Co., 1996.

Dossey, Larry. *Healing Words*. New York: HarperCollins, 1993.

Dossey, Larry. *Recovering the Soul*. New York: Bantam, 1989.

Easwaran, Eknath (trans). *The Baghavad Gita*. Tomales, California: Nilgiri Press, 1996.

In Dire Straits

Frankl, Victor. *The Unheard Cry for Meaning*. New York: Washington Square Press, 1984.

Golan, Ralph. *Optimum Wellness*, New York: Ballantine Books, 1999.

Goleman, Daniel. *Vital Lies, Simple Truths*. New York: Simon and Schuster, 1985.

Goswami, Amit. *The Self-Aware Universe—How Consciousness Creates the Material World*. Los Angeles: Tarcher, 1993.

Greenberg, Michael. *Paradox and Healing*. Victoria, Canada: Meridian House, 1992.

Grof, Christina. *The Thirst for Wholeness—Attachment, Addiction and the Spiritual Path*. San Francisco: HarperSanFrancisco, 1993.

Gould, Stephen Jay. *The Panda's Thumb*. New York: W.W. Norton and Company, 1980.

Hanh, Thich Nhat. *Peace in Every Step: The Path of Mindfulness in Everyday Life*. New York: Bantam, 1991.

Harman, Willis. *Higher Creativity—Liberating the Unconscious for Breakthrough Insights*. Los Angeles: Tarcher, 1984.

Hesse, Herman. *Siddhartha*. New York: Bantam, 1971.

Hixson, Lex. *Coming Home*. Burdett, New York: Larson Publications, 1978.

Hughes, Robert. *The Shock of the New*. New York: Alfred A. Knopf, 1982.

Joy, W. Brugh. *Joy's Way*. Los Angeles: Tarcher, 1979.

Kabat-Zinn, Jon. *Full Catastrophe Living*. New York: Dell Publishing, 1990.

Kidd, Sue Monk. *The Secret Life of Bees*. New York: Penguin

Books, 2002.

Kopp, Sheldon. *Guru—Metaphors from a Psychotherapist*. Palo Alto, California: Science and Behavior Books, 1971.

Kopp, Sheldon. *If You Meet the Buddha on the Road, Kill Him*. New York: Bantam, 1972.

Kopp, Sheldon. *Raise Your Right Hand Against Fear*. Minneapolis, MN: ComCare Publishers, 1988.

Kornfield, Jack. *A Path with Heart*. New York: Bantam, 1993.

Kuhn, Thomas S. *The Structure of Scientific Revolution*. Chicago: University of Chicago Press, 1962.

Kumar, Satish. *Path Without Destination*. New York: William Morrow, 1972.

Lama Surya Das. *Awakening to the Sacred*. New York: Broadway Books, 1999.

Lama Surya Das. *Awakening the Buddha Within*. New York: Broadway Books, 1997.

Levine, Steven. *Who Dies*. New York: Doubleday, 1982.

Lowen, M.D., Alexander. *The Spirituality of the Body*. New York: MacMillan, 1990.

May, Rollo. *The Courage to Create*. New York: Bantam, 1976.

Miller, Henry. *The Paintings of Henry Miller—Paint as You Like and Die Happy*. New York: Chronicle Books, 1973.

Miller, Henry. *Stand Still Like the Hummingbird*. New York: New Directions, 1962.

Murphy, Michael. *The Future of the Body*. Los Angeles: Tarcher, 1992.

Peat, F. David. *Synchronicity—The Bridge Between Matter and Mind*. New York: Bantam, 1988.

Pierrakos, Eva. *The Pathwork of Self-Transformation*. New York: Bantam, 1990.

Rinpoche, Sogyal. *The Tibetan book of Living and Dying*. San Francisco: HarperSanFrancisco, 1994.

Rothschild, Joel. *Signals*. California: New World Library, 2001.

Samuels, M.D., Mike. Bennett, Hal Zina, *Well Body Well Earth*. San Francisco: Sierra Club Books, 1985.

Scammell, Henry. *The New Arthritis Breakthrough*. New York: M. Evans and Company, Inc., 1993.

Scammell, Henry. *Scleroderma*. New York: M. Evans and Company, Inc., 1988,

Shainberg, Lawrence. *Ambivalent Zen*. New York: Vintage Books, 1955.

Sheehan, George. *This Running Life*. New York: Fireside Book, 1980.

Sheldrake, Rupert. *Dogs That Know When Their Owners are Coming Home*. New York: Three Rivers Press, 1999.

Sheldrake, Rupert. *Presence of the Past*. Rochester, Vermont: Park Street Press, 1988.

Siegel, Bernie. *Love Medicine and Miracles*. New York: Harper and Row Publishers, 1986.

Talbott, Michael. *The Holographic Universe*. New York: Harper Perennial, 1991.

Walsh, Roger and Vaughn, Francis, Editors. *Paths Beyond Ego, The Transpersonal Vision*. Los Angeles: Tarcher, 1993.

Watts, Alan. *The Way of Liberation*. New York: Weatherhill Press, 1983.

Welch, Holmes. *Taoism—The Parting of the Way*. Boston: Beacon Press, 1957.

Welwood, John. *Journey of the Heart*. New York: Harper Perennial, 1990.

Wilber, Ken. *Grace and Grit*. Boston: Shambhala, 1991.

Wilber, Ken. *Sex Ecology and Spirituality*. Boston: Shambhala, 1995.

Wilson, E.O., *The Creation, An Appeal to Save Life on Earth*. W. W. Norton & Company, 2006.

Zinn, Howard. *A People's History of the United States*. New York: HarperCollins, 1980.

Zukav, Gary. *The Seat of the Soul*. New York: Simon and Schuster, 1989.

In Dire Straits

Index

In Dire Straits

In Dire Straits

Mass Extinctions, Wilson, E.O., 200; also see Sydney's Thumb and Climate Change

Miller, Henry, 163

Mindful Travel and Disease, the book, 9, 45; Buddhism 6; enlightened warrior, 13, 92, 100, 104, 106, 117; explorer mentality, 4, 87; grief, 45; impediments and resourcefulness, 4–6, 7; mystic, 92–93; travel at home, 12, 52

Non-locality, 146–148, 181; also see Consciousness and Healing and Sheldrake, Rupert

Optimal Wellness, cohealing, 19, 199; leaky gut 31; pathways 16; stressors, 24

Pharmaceutical Companies, 59; also see Brown, Thomas M.

Psoriatic Arthritis, 9, 26, 28, 51, 55, 66, 80, 85, 86, 130, 170, 187, 190

Radical Ideas, 19–22; Kopp, Sheldon 22

Satya, 101, writing and exposing the truth, 106–107, 116–117, 128–129; also see Mindful Travel at http://www.SydneysThumb.com

Sheldrake, Rupert, animal intuition, 151; morphic fields and non-locality, 145

Ship of Fools, 132–138

Siddhis, 179

Staring Into the Abyss, 139

In Dire Straits

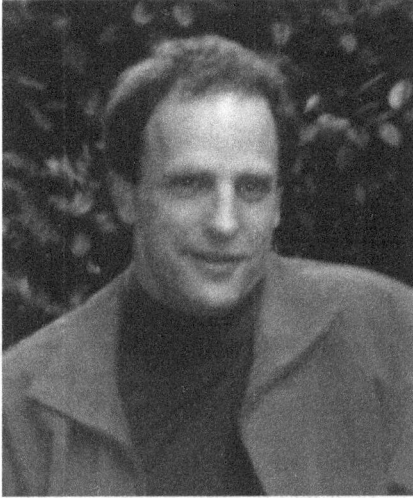

About the Author

Jim Currie is a Seattle writer and ecologist whose credits include works of fiction, non-fiction, and over twenty publications on natural resource management and biology. He holds an honor's degree from Harvard and a masters from Berkeley. His writing and teaching reflect an interdisciplinary perspective and wide-ranging curiosity in the arts, science, humanities and philosophy.

His published titles include "The Mindful Traveler: A Guide to Journaling and Transformative Travel" (Open Court, 2000). His work in the environmental field includes innovative ways to protect water quality and habitat. His teaching and lecturing draw upon integral psychology and Eastern philosophy.

Jim writes extensively on ecology, conservation and sustainable economy. His web-based organization at

http://www.SydneysThumb.com

includes members from across the globe and is dedicated to climate action, species rescue and travel that leaves shallow footprints.

If you enjoyed *In Dire Straits* consider these other fine Books from Savant Books and Publications:

A Whale's Tale by Daniel S. Janik
Tropic *of California* by R. Page Kaufman
The Village Curtain by Tony Tame
Dare to Love in Oz by William Maltese
The Interzone by Tasuyuki Kobayashi
Today I Am A Man by Larry Rodness
The Bahrain Conspiracy by Bentley Gates
Called Home by Gloria Schumann
Kanaka Blues by Mike Farris
First Breath: 2010 Savant Anthology of Poems Z. Oliver (Ed)
Poor Rich by Jean Blasiar
The *Jumper Chronicles* by W. C. Peever
William Maltese's Flicker by William Maltese
My Unborn Child by Orest Stocco
Perilous Panacea by Ronald Klueh
Last Song of the Whales by Four Arrows
Falling but Fulfilled by Zachary M. Oliver
Still Life with Cat and Mouse by Sheila McGraw
Manifest Intent by Mike Farris
Mythical Voyage by Robin Ymer
Hello, Norm Jean by Sue Dolleris
Richer by Jean Blasiar
Charlie No Face by David B. Seaburn
Number One Bestseller by Brian Morley

Scheduled for Release in 2011:
Ammon's Horn by Guerrino Amati
In the Himalayan Nights by Anoop Chandola
Blood Money by Scott Mastro
The Treasure of La Escondida by Carolyn Kingson
Wretched Land by Mila Komarnisky
Chan Kim by Ilan Herman

http://www.savantbooksandpublications.com

www.ingramcontent.com/pod-product-compliance
Lightning Source LLC
Chambersburg PA
CBHW072123270326
41931CB00010B/1651